WHAT YOU NEED TO KNOW ABOUT MENOPAUSE

What You Need to Know about Menopause

Dr. Paul Reisser
and Teri Reisser

VINE
BOOKS

Servant Publications
Ann Arbor, Michigan

Vine Books is an imprint of Servant Publications especially
designed to serve evangelical Christians.

Published by Servant Publications
P.O. Box 8617
Ann Arbor, Michigan 48107

Cover design by Syncom
94 95 96 97 98 10 9 8 7 6 5 4 3 2 1

Printed in the United States of America
ISBN 0-89283-880-9

Contents

ACKNOWLEDGMENTS

We would like to thank the following people for their various roles in helping us complete this project:

Teri's mother, Wanda Ketchum, and a number of her friends who were willing to be transparent in discussing their menopausal experiences.

Paul's parents, Don and Harriet Reisser, for unending support and for those wonderful, weekly family dinners which have provided so much respite and relaxation.

Our children, Chad and Carrie, who were both helpful and patient during the intensive final weeks of preparing the manuscript.

Our long-suffering editor, Cindy Maddox, for so many excellent suggestions and fine-tunings.

INTRODUCTION

Why should I read this? Introductions are almost as boring as acknowledgments.

We know that introductory material can get a little dull, but there's some important stuff here, so please listen up.

First and foremost, we have tried throughout this project to avoid some of the dryness that can creep into a health-related book—especially one about menopause. To help move things along, we decided to use a question and answer format, but one that's more like a dialogue than a medical catechism. And our assumption is that the questions are coming from someone who didn't just fall off the turnip truck.

Good idea—I hate being talked down to.

We'll try to avoid any patronizing, although we do reserve the right to throw in a few pep talks and an occasional tirade. But you also need to hear some disclaimers before we proceed.

Here it comes ... the old "See your doctor first" routine, right?

Well, yes. In a book, it's impossible to take into account the uniqueness of each individual's life and circumstances.

9

Some information is universally applicable—for example, the infinite wisdom of quitting smoking. But most medical decisions, especially if they involve a prescription or two, need an appropriate history and physical exam before proceeding. Also, as medical research on menopause and related subjects continues to forge ahead, what you read today may be subject to some revision next year.

You should also know that this book is not meant to be a medical encyclopedia. Our objective has been to review the overall sweep of the menopausal process, with an emphasis (believe it or not) on the positive. We think it's more important to understand, and hopefully put into use, a few basic but important ideas rather than be swamped by an avalanche of details.

Anything else before I fall asleep or flip ahead to the chapter on sex?

One final note on our basic perspective. Medically, we have tried to stay in the middle of the road. If you want the latest news from the fringes or a compendium of alternative therapies, this book isn't for you. And, speaking of sex, we have made no secret of our esteem for the biblical viewpoint on that topic and all others as well. While many contemporary books written for women seem to relegate marriage, family, and traditional values to the dust pile of history, we believe they should be promoted and defended vigorously. But we are also enthusiastic proponents of a woman making the most of her life and expanding her horizons at whatever age or stage she finds herself. We don't believe that one ideal must be sacrificed for the other.

Sounds good to me. Can I move on now?

Yes, you may. And we hope you enjoy the trip.

Chapter One

ﾟ∞∞ﾟ

Who Wants to Read about Aging?

When we began doing research for this book, Teri approached some of her mother's friends (ages forty-six to seventy) to see if they would be willing to sit down over coffee and talk freely about their menopausal experiences. The unanimous response was, "You're *kidding!*" Although these women had known each other for years, the group got off to an awkward start. We became increasingly aware that this episode of life, though universal among women, has seldom been a popular discussion topic.

Why have women traditionally been so reluctant to talk about menopause?

A combination of physical factors, embarrassment, negative mythology, and outright dread have kept women silent on this subject for decades. Only for the past two or three generations have a majority of women lived long enough to *reach* menopause, much less *discuss* it. At the turn of the century, the average female life expectancy was a whopping forty-nine years, while women in developed countries today live an average of eighty years. One reason the menopausal process has been shrouded in mystery is *not* because of the previous generation's Victorian prudishness, but because there simply hasn't been hundreds of years of wisdom passed down from mother to daughter.

But this is only part of the problem. Western culture is obsessed with youth and good looks, especially among women. With desirability and value tied so closely to beauty rather than more enduring attributes, menopause has carried some massively negative baggage: visions of wrinkles, graying, infirmity, and (even worse) depression, isolation, and impending mortality. Too many people have seen menopause as the internal signal of the beginning of the end—the downhill slide, membership in the "over the hill gang."

In addition, women haven't always received much aid and comfort at the doctor's office. Physician's attitudes toward the concerns and complaints of women at mid-life and beyond have not been exactly enthusiastic, especially when the patient's list of symptoms has been lengthy and the visit time cramped. A pat on the head and a prescription for tranquilizers was all too often the bottom line in these interactions. In addition, for decades the vast majority of doctors caring exclusively for women have been men. Gender, of course, does not determine quality of care, but it can affect how seriously certain issues are addressed.

Only recently has medical literature taken an earnest interest in women's health issues (other than those strictly related to reproduction). In a huge "better late than never" project, the National Institute of Health is undertaking a study called the Women's Health Initiative. This will attempt to address in a definitive way some probable links between diet and cancer, hormones and heart disease, and calcium/Vitamin D and osteoporosis (thinning of the bones).

So why am I seeing more books on the shelves about menopause now—including this one?

Three reasons. First, for all of its excesses and its hostility to many traditional values, the feminist movement has brought before the public the important notion that women are not mere appendages to men but have capabilities extending far beyond decorative and reproductive functions. Raising expectations for life and significance beyond the fertile years has been an important by-product of this movement.

Second, Baby Boomers are just now entering menopause with a vengeance. There are more than fifty-two million women over age forty in this country today, and that number is rapidly growing. (Comic Dave Barry has quipped that this number of women experiencing simultaneous hot flashes could seriously impact global warming by the turn of the century.) This generation has grown up being the center of national attention. Pumped up by Ralph Nader and assertiveness training classes, the Boomers are clearly not willing to settle for the ambiguity that has traditionally shrouded the menopausal process.

Third, many women in the Christian community are open to discussing the full length and breadth of life issues. This important contingent of American society brings the added dimension of a desire to serve God and experience his abundance through the entire course of life. One need not be a radical feminist to deal directly and frankly with the facts of reproductive physiology, with medical issues, and with long-term decisions affecting quality and direction of life.

Okay, I'm a "Baby Boomer"—so educate me! What exactly is "menopause"?

Strictly speaking, the term *menopause* does not refer to a process but simply to the very last menstrual cycle of a women's reproductive life. *Perimenopause* refers specifically to the transitional period of time between normal reproductive cycles and the final menstrual flow; likewise, *postmenopause* refers to the years following the last period. *Climacteric* is a less commonly used term which designates the entire process spanning roughly five years before and after menopause. For the sake of simplicity, we will use the word *menopause* to refer to the entire transitional time surrounding the end of menses. (Actually, most people find the word *climacteric* a bit obscure, and we got tired of typing out *perimenopause*.)

What happens during menopause?

As we will discuss in more detail in the next chapter, menopause is the process during which a woman's reproductive cycles end. When a woman approaches her fifties (and sometimes earlier), the ovaries' supply of eggs (or ova) become depleted. At the same time, they begin to reduce their production of estrogen and progesterone, the hormones which prepare the uterus for implantation of a fertilized egg. Essentially, the ovaries "retire" from their thirty- to forty-year career of egg and hormone supply (though lesser amounts of various hormones are still manufactured). This may occur rapidly or over several years, during which a number of important physical and emotional changes occur in a woman—not the least of which is her loss of fertility.

When can I expect menopause and how long will this charming process affect me?

Do we sense a little hostility? Remember: menopause is not a disease. It is a universal event in the human female, but its individual impact varies greatly. It may occur without notice, or it may produce disruptive symptoms. It may generate little in the way of long-term consequences, or its ultimate effect on the course of life may be profound.

The vast majority of women experience menopause between the ages of forty-five and fifty-five, with the average

age currently fifty-one. Of course, some women will enter the process before age forty, some as late as sixty. Teri's own mom started at age thirty-three and was finished two years later. There doesn't seem to be any relationship between the age at which a woman begins her periods and the timing of menopause. Nor does the age of onset appear to be affected by race, marital status, or geography. Smokers, however, experience menopause nearly two years earlier than nonsmokers. And women who have had ovaries removed surgically during their reproductive years have, by definition, an abrupt menopause.

The cessation of menstrual cycles is usually gradual, marked by increasing length of cycles: 70 percent of all women will experience such irregularity, with thirty-six to ninety days between periods. In contrast, 10 percent will experience an abrupt end to their periods without warning. Another 18 percent report *more* bleeding than usual. This may reflect a problem with the lining of the uterus, however, and should be evaluated by a physician.

To demonstrate the variability of this whole phenomenon, none of the women interviewed for this book fit this description of "average" onset and duration!

Do men go through a form of menopause, or is this just special treatment for the ladies?

From a reproductive standpoint (and some would say many other ways as well) men are much less complex than women. Rather than experiencing the intricate interplay of hormones which characterizes the female cycle, the male testes crank out sperm and the hormone testosterone (and an array of others known in general as "androgens") more or less constantly after puberty. Production of both sperm and testosterone tend to decline slowly during a man's later years, and a variety of medical and psychological problems can affect his sexual function.

Some authors, especially in Europe, have used the term *andropause* to refer to this gradual decline of male hormonal function, along with a collection of emotional and personal events associated with mid-life. The concept of a male menopause has mostly been fueled by behavior, especially the infamous "middle-age crazy" sports car and spouse-dumping passages, or less flamboyant mid-life re-evaluations. But there is no universal event marking the end of male reproduction, and some gentlemen even in their eighth and ninth decades have sired children.

Interestingly, men produce small amounts of estrogen (just as females make a certain amount of their own androgens), and their estrogen levels increase 50 percent between age twenty-five and fifty while testosterone is decreasing. (Perhaps this is why many men mellow out and become more lovable as they age!) There is, to be sure, no recommendation for widespread testosterone replacement in this age group, though some with overt failure of the testes can benefit, provided they are monitored for prostate cancer. Thus, men must muddle through their mid-life changes without any overtly helpful hormonal therapy.

Back to me... what exactly can I look forward to during this multi-year process?

You may be one of the blessed few who don't experience much at all. Or you may find yourself contending with all of those nasty symptoms you've heard about (whispered with rolling eyes and clucking tongues): hot flashes, night sweats, skin and hair changes, sudden irritability, tingling sensations, sleep disturbances, vaginal dryness, vaginal odor, lessening of sexual desire—are we having fun yet? And whether or not you experience these acute symptoms, you will need to think about, plan for, and deal with long term issues: maintaining the best possible heart and lung function, screening for unsuspected disease, preserving the bones, and making decisions about hormone replacement therapy.

Good grief! With a list like that, I think I'll just forget and hope for the best! Why on earth would I want to read about all these unpleasant events?

For the same reason women go through birth classes prior to delivery: because knowledge dispels fear. Just as the pains of childbirth are made more manageable by understanding and working *with* the process of labor, so the physical and emotional turmoil of menopause can be minimized by foreknowledge and planning for this important period of your life.

Many women merrily approach the menopausal process as if denial of its existence means it won't happen to them—especially if their periods, pregnancies, and childbirths have been relatively uncomplicated. Unfortunately, the tired old stereotype of postmenopausal women as depressed, hypochondriachal dowagers makes the whole process look like something the rest of us would just as soon skip, thank you very much!

This book is meant to be a wake-up call. We will certainly address the physical components of menopause in some depth. But there are some equally important concerns—personal, emotional, vocational, and spiritual issues—which are affected by menopause. The mental and spiritual attitudes with which you enter this process can greatly influence the direction of the entire experience.

Specifically, we hope to motivate you to:

1. Learn about the events that are going to happen to you (whether you like them or not).
2. Adopt some very basic lifestyle habits—a "Maintenance

Checklist"—that will prevent a host of physical and emotional problems.

3. Go through the appropriate medical hassles that screen for diseases that can sneak up on you.

4. Make an informed decision about whether to take certain steps, including hormone replacement, to deal with the specific effects of estrogen loss.

5. See the midlife years and beyond as a time of great opportunity for personal and spiritual growth, achievement, and service to God.

Ultimately, only you can make the physical and emotional preparations that will ensure a smoother transition than the one your mother may have experienced. But we hope we can convince you that you don't need or want menopause to take you by surprise.

You make this sound like a ride at Disneyland. Be serious! Isn't it pretty much downhill once you enter the menopausal process?

Only if you *choose* to take a downhill direction! Remember: the average woman will live for *thirty years after menopause*. Women who are currently between the ages of forty-five and sixty are completely rewriting the script for middle age. Whereas their mothers felt old at fifty-five or sixty, it is increasingly common for postmenopausal women to start whole new careers. This is an unprecedented time in the history of womankind, and it presents the unique opportunity to redefine middle and old age and to create new role models for the generations to follow.

For the first time, women are beginning to view menopause as a natural event and not something to be ashamed of. With the kind of information we now possess about preparing for and managing the events surrounding menopause, there is *no reason* to cling to the tired notion that hot flashes signal

the beginning of a life spent in emotional upheaval, or vege-
tating in an old rocker on the back porch! With the busy years
of childrearing behind, with the fantasy of eternal youthful
looks happily abandoned, the postmenopausal years can truly
be the most creative and fulfilling period of a woman's entire
life.

Chapter Two

⚬⚬⚬

What's Going On (or Off) at Menopause?

As we mentioned in the first chapter, *menopause* technically designates the end of menstrual cycles. But like most events in the human body, this is a visible milestone in an important process that has been taking place for some time. It isn't the sudden flipping of a biological switch.

Is the main event in menopause a change in the uterus itself?

Not really—it is only doing what it's told. The uterus, of course, is extremely important as the place where the fertilized egg implants and then hopefully continues developing until a child is born. But its status, and in particular the ebb and flow of its delicate inner lining (known as the endometrium), is governed primarily by estrogen and progesterone, two important hormones manufactured by the ovaries. The production of these hormones occurs under the direction of the pituitary gland situated at the base of the brain. And the pituitary takes orders from the hypothalamus, directly above it.

Hang on—do I really need to know a lot of complicated biology to understand why menstrual periods stop?

You don't need to know every excruciating detail. But in order to make some important decisions, it does help to understand who's doing what and why. For now, think of the monthly cycle as an elegant, four-tiered system with an overriding purpose: bringing a new human being into the world.

Starting from the top, the hypothalamus (which also regulates such important functions as hunger, thirst, and temperature) begins each cycle by sending a hormonal message to the pituitary gland, in the form of a protein which has been dubbed *gonadotrophic releasing hormone,* or GRH.

Could you give me a simple definition of a hormone?

Basically, a hormone is a biochemical message sent from one part of the body through the bloodstream to one or more target organs, with a very specific set of effects. While we tend to think of hormones as being primarily involved in sexual functions, many bodily functions are influenced by hormonal compounds. Insulin, for example, is a hormone necessary to escort glucose into cells, and the thyroid hormone regulates the metabolic rate of the entire system.

OK, so GRH travels to the pituitary, right?

Very good. This tiny structure hangs like a pea-sized punching bag from the brain, protected by a bony enclosure. Years ago the pituitary was named the *master gland* because its hormones stimulate the thyroid and adrenal glands, the ovaries in women and testes in men, and the production of milk after the birth of a child. In response to GRH in a woman, the pituitary produces *follicle stimulating hormone,* or or FSH. This causes a number of ova to begin ripening within the ovary. (The term ova refers to the *oocytes,* or egg cells, large single cells which contain half of the genetic code of a human being. The sperm cells of the male also contain half of the genetic code. The combining of the codes when sperm and egg unite is known as fertilization, the first moment of human life.)

I thought that, in general, only one egg was produced by the ovary every month.

Basically, that is true. The ovaries, which lie adjacent to the uterus in the pelvis, already contain all of the eggs a woman will ever have in her lifetime—about 500,000 at birth. (During fetal development, a female begins with many times that number.) Every month, under the influence of FSH, several eggs begin the process, but only one is actually "chosen" to complete a developmental cycle that was arrested prior to birth. Of this initial stash of a half million cells, only between three hundred and four hundred will fully ripen and exit the ovary over the course of a woman's reproductive life.

As that egg continues to ripen, a tiny sac of fluid surrounding it, known as a follicle, enlarges, and cells lining the follicle begin secreting increasing levels of estrogen. (Hence the naming of the pituitary's messenger as "follicle stimulating hormone....") Estrogen stimulates the uterus to begin building up its inner lining, the endometrium—the first stage of its preparation for a possible pregnancy.

What happens next?

About two weeks into the cycle, the rising levels of estrogen also trigger the pituitary to fire off a "surge" of another hormone known as *luteinizing hormone* (or LH for short).

Wait a minute. I thought the pituitary told the ovaries what to do, not the other way around.

Actually, many hormone systems operate with what is called a "feedback loop," where the target organ's response influences the behavior of the sender of the hormonal message. To illustrate the point, compare this to sending your child a message to clean his room. Your child responds, "When I get around to it"—which triggers your response, "Then you'll get your allowance when *I* get around to it." In any event, the LH surge boots the ripened egg out of the ovary, a process called ovulation. Some women can feel this occurring, and some actually experience a pain called *mittelschmerz* (German for "middle pain") every month when this takes place.

What determines which ovary sends an egg on its way?

Good question. The process appears to be random since there is no pattern determining whether the right or left side provides the monthly egg.

What happens to the other eggs that were stimulated but not fully ripened?

They atrophy, or literally disappear from the ovarian tissue. This is a true example of a situation in which "many are called but few are chosen." Of course, in some situations, more than one egg ovulates during a given cycle, resulting in twins, triplets, and so forth.

What happens to the egg that is chosen?

If everything is working properly, it is plucked from the

ovary by tentacle-like structures extending from the end of a nearby conduit called the fallopian tube. This gently carries the egg on a brief journey to the uterus. If the egg happens to encounter some sperm sprinting upstream through the tube, and one of those sperm plows into the egg and injects its genetic material—and if all goes according to plan—a new human being will appear nine months later.

Meanwhile, back at the ovary, LH transforms the vacant follicle into a structure called the corpus luteum (literally "yellow body"). LH luteinizing hormone, is named in honor of this function. The corpus luteum becomes a factory for progesterone, which completes the preparation of the lining of the uterus. Dr. Wulf Utian, a prominent menopause researcher, has likened estrogen to a contractor which carries out the basic construction inside the uterus, while progesterone is the "interior decorator" which does the finish work.

If the egg is fertilized and successfully implants in the uterus, it immediately begins to produce its own progesterone supply, since this hormone is absolutely necessary to maintain the endometrium (and thus the pregnancy). But if fertilization does not occur, the egg passes through the uterus. The corpus luteum runs out of steam and stops producing progesterone. Without the progesterone support, the lining of the uterus deteriorates and exits the uterus as a flow of tissue and blood we call the menstrual period.

The terms *menstrual*, and *menses*, and *menopause* all derive from the Latin *mensis*, which means, appropriately enough, "month." Indeed, the prototype cycle is about every twenty-eight days, although that number may vary from twenty-one to thirty-five days in healthy women. Interestingly, the variability arises only in the first half of the cycle. Once the egg has started its journey, a rather precise biological stopwatch has been started: virtually without exception, the time from ovulation to menstrual flow is fourteen days.

So what happens at menopause? Does the ovary run out of eggs?

Actually, a number of changes occur in the ovary. The number of eggs is indeed depleted over the thirty to forty years when a woman is capable of reproducing, until about ten thousand are left at the time of menopause. More significantly, the follicles become less sensitive to the pituitary's FSH message. They may produce some estrogen but not complete the process of ovulation, causing the uterus to receive some stimulation but without the progesterone finish work. Menstrual bleeding may thus become erratic. Furthermore, if the endometrium becomes overly stimulated, the thicker lining cannot be sustained and bleeding may be much heavier.

Finally, the follicles become completely unresponsive to FSH. Estrogen and progesterone levels decline but don't completely disappear.

Why is that?

A low level of hormones continues to exit the ovaries even after the monthly cycles end. Furthermore, some estrogen is created in the adrenal glands and in fatty tissue all over the body. In fact, women with an ample supply of fat may generate enough estrogen to minimize the symptoms that thinner women experience when their estrogen levels fall. This is no great benefit, however, because of the many other drawbacks of obesity—one of which is, ironically, increased risk of cancer of the uterus, arising from relentless stimulation of the endometrium by the higher estrogen levels.

Does the pituitary stop making FSH when the ovaries have slowed down their estrogen production?

No, it doesn't. In fact, neither the hypothalamus nor the pituitary seem terribly bright in this regard. In what appears to be an effort to get the ovaries' attention, they crank out high levels of GRH, FSH, and LH to no avail. Indeed, measuring FSH in the bloodstream serves as a useful confirmation that menopause has occurred. Interestingly, the hypothalamus and pituitary never give up; even the most aged woman will be found to have very high FSH levels.

So basically, the organ that is the center of attraction at menopause is the ovary, right?

Correct. These egg and hormone factories retire, signaling the end of reproduction—but not the end of a fruitful life. There is no getting around this event and for good reason: given the rigors of childbirth and the length of time required to raise a newborn to near-adulthood, it would be unwise (with extremely rare exceptions) for a woman to become pregnant after age sixty.

Paul has one patient who has been seeing a "nutritionist" who claims that special dietary supplements will prevent menopause from occurring. Unfortunately, both she and her delusional advisor have the mistaken notion that menopause is a disease. For some reason, medical literature has had a tendency until recently to view almost every aspect of female reproduction as a disorder of some sort. (Even now, some abortion clinics advertise their services as "pregnancy resolution," as if it too were a disease.) Menopause is a universal process with certain consequences which in many cases can create distress or contribute to other complications. But it is not a pathology to be cured.

Does estrogen serve any function beyond preparing the uterus for pregnancy?

Indeed, it does. Most of the events of puberty occur as a result of an increase in estrogen production by the ovaries, which are set in motion by signals from the hypothalamus and pituitary in response to an internal "wake-up call." Estrogen sets off a pre-pubertal growth spurt, and then stimulates growth and development of the breasts, external genitalia, vagina, and fallopian tubes as a girl passes into adulthood. Throughout the reproductive years, estrogen serves in a supporting role for these organs, as well as for the urinary tract and skin. Furthermore, as we will explore later, estrogen helps prevent bone loss and reduces the risk for coronary artery disease.

Actually, to be completely accurate, we should note that the term *estrogen* designates a collection of compounds produced by your body which have estrogenic activity. These are estradiol, a potent form produced primarily by the ovary which fluctuates with the monthly cycle; estrone, which is produced mainly outside of the ovary; and estriol, a weaker form which is considered primarily to be a metabolic product of the others. Unless otherwise noted, we will use the single term *estrogen* to designate all of these hormones as a group.

So what happens when the estrogen levels drop?

Several changes in the peri- and postmenopausal woman are attributes to the decline of this important hormone.

1. Irregular menses. One of the most important signals that the perimenopausal years may have arrived is the onset of irregular menstrual cycles. The variations on this theme are numerous and can change depending on the production of estrogen from the ovaries, as well as whether or not an egg has been produced each month. For example, a low output of estrogen causes little stimulation for the lining of the uterus to grow, and so the menstrual flow may be scant. On the other hand, if ovulation doesn't occur, the progesterone "ripening" of the uterus won't either. This may lead to a steady buildup of endometrial lining in the uterus, which sloughs in bits and pieces (producing spotting) or a veritable flood of tissue all at once.

So there's no sure-fire way to tell from the flow pattern that menopause is imminent?

That's right. The cycles may occur farther apart or closer together, and they may be heavier or lighter than usual. Interestingly, some women develop a pronounced premenstrual irritability during the perimenopause, often to their dismay—and their family's as well. This "late onset PMS" is not a sign that a woman is falling apart at the seams, but is a genuine (if intense) response to hormonal variations. In *Man - aging Your Menopause,* Dr. Wulf Utian uses the term *pre-menopausal syndrome* to characterize women who rarely have PMS symptoms in the early reproductive years but develop them later on (Prentiss Hall Press, 1990).

Are there any menstrual flow patterns I should be concerned about?

In general, a shift toward greater menstrual flows—whether prolonged in length or very heavy for the usual number of days or both—deserves some attention. While this may indeed reflect a perimenopausal change in hormonal blend, it might also be caused by *hyperplasia,* a worrisome buildup of the uterine lining which might progress to cancer, or even worse, an overt cancer of this tissue. Fibroids, which are benign muscular growths in the uterus, can also cause heavy bleeding. Less common, but no less important, are assorted problems such as clotting disorders or thyroid disease. In addition, the ongoing blood loss can outstrip the body's capacity to replace red cells, deplete iron stores, and lead to iron deficiency anemia—which, fortunately, is readily correctable, but a clear indication that bleeding is excessive.

What should I do if I'm concerned about heavy bleeding?

For two or three cycles, keep track of the number of days you bleed, how heavy the flow appears to be (gauged by the number of pads or tampons you need to stay ahead of it), and how many days elapse between cycles. Then review the situation with your primary care physician or gynecologist. When all is said and done, you may need an endometrial biopsy (an office procedure) or a full-blown D & C to make sure nothing serious is happening. (D & C is short for *dilatation and curettage*, a procedure in the operating room under anesthesia which scrapes out the endometrial lining and sends it to the pathologist to be evaluated.)

Is there anything to be concerned about if I skip periods?

This is a common pattern for perimenopausal women, with the distance between cycles increasing until they finally stop altogether. The most significant alternative explanation to rule out, believe it or not, would be pregnancy.

Even for a woman in her forties?

Or beyond. As long as eggs are traveling down the fallopian tubes and sperm are there to meet them, a pregnancy can begin. If there's any such possibility, check it out: and if you have questions about that possibility, don't hesitate to bring it up with your doctor, who may not be thinking along those lines.

2. Hot flashes. These well-known annoyances occur in at least 75 percent of menopausal women. They typically involve a sensation of heat rising from the chest toward the face and arms, accompanied by flushing of the skin, and less often by an increased heart rate and overt sweating. They may occur once in a while or several times a day and last anywhere from a few minutes to a half hour.

Needless to say, these can be extremely annoying. A woman that Teri interviewed told this story: "One time I was coming home from church, and I was so hot I thought I was going to have a stroke. So I took off my blouse and was driving down the boulevard in my bra, praying no one would see me!" Another woman described a distressing situation when she was standing during a crowded meeting and a hot flash suddenly came on: "It was like the dye they put in your veins for a venogram—you just start feeling this flush all over. I thought I was going to scream and start ripping my clothes off right then and there!" (Incidentally, we don't recommend *stripping* as a response to hot flashes—particularly if you happen to be in public!)

What causes these delightful episodes?

They appear to be associated with sudden changes in estrogen levels, which in turn trigger an overzealous response from the hypothalamus. Remember that this area of the brain starts the monthly cycle, and later tries in vain to get things going after the ovaries sign off. The hypothalamus also regulates body temperature and other primal functions, partly through changes in blood vessel diameter, and apparently it sends an overabundance of messages to the circulatory system in response to the fluctuation of estrogen.

How long does this go on, and what can be done about it?

Fortunately, the hypothalamus eventually adjusts to the change in the hormonal environment and calms down, although the process may take a few months or a few years. For those who take estrogen replacement, disruptive flashes and flushes quickly come to an end, as will be discussed in Chapter Six. For those who do not opt for hormone replacement, an effort to identify hot flash "triggers" and then avoid them, can pay off. These triggers might include certain foods, especially spicy dishes, caffeine, alcohol, and even sugar; rapid changes in temperature, such as entering a chilled office building on a hot summer day; and stressful situations which provoke the autonomic nervous system into action.

In addition, a variety of medications have been proposed over the years to quiet flushes and flashes, although none can be considered an overwhelming success. Progesterone, for example, appears to help, but there are very few situations in which one would want this hormone supplemented by itself. (Among other things, it has an anti-estrogenic effect which the rest of the anatomy will not appreciate.) Certain medications which lower blood pressure by stabilizing small blood vessels have seen limited service in the hot flash war, although they have their own list of potential side effects. One of the most widely used non-estrogen treatments for hot flashes has been Bellergal, a grab-bag of autonomic nervous system calmers combined with a little phenobarbital. For some women this concoction seems to work extremely well, although a physician should review several items before this prescription goes to the pharmacist.

3. Vaginal atrophy. The vagina is extremely sensitive to estrogen stimulation, and without it the vagina undergoes a number of changes. The mucus membranes which line it become thinner, and its secretions become less abundant and less acidic. The vagina also becomes shorter and narrower. Irritation, itching, and burning may result, a condition known as atrophic vaginitis. Needless to say, these developments may make sexual intercourse increasingly uncomfortable, if not downright impossible. (More on this in Chapter Eight.)

4. Urinary tract problems. The cells that line the bladder and urethra (the short tube connecting the bladder to the outside world), and the muscular layers of these structures, become thinner after estrogen levels decline. This may lead to difficulty controlling the release of urine (incontinence), a sensation of needing to void more often (known as frequency), and burning with the passage of urine (called dysuria). In addition, these changes reduce the normal defenses against any bacteria which happen to wander by, and many postmenopausal women are thus plagued by repeated bladder infections.

How would I tell the difference between bladder symptoms needing estrogen and those needing antibiotics?

Good question. The symptoms are so similar that, if and when they show up, the urine should be checked and possibly cultured to clarify whether one or both are the problem. Furthermore, loss of muscle tone in the pelvis may lead to stress incontinence, an annoying loss of urine with anything that increases pressure in the abdomen (such as coughing, sneezing, or laughing). Stress incontinence is less a hormonal than a mechanical problem, which may be improved by Kegel exercises (see Chapter Eight) but may require surgery to correct disruptive symptoms which aren't responding to more conservative measures.

5. Skin changes. Both layers of skin—the epidermis and dermis—are sensitive to estrogen support. At the surface, estrogen promotes lubrication and water retention. In the deeper dermis, estrogen stimulates production of collagen, a protein that maintains thickness and elasticity of skin. As a result, declining estrogen levels accelerate the thinning, drying, and wrinkling of skin.

I notice that women who take estrogen aren't immune to developing wrinkles. Aren't there other factors which age the skin?

If estrogen replacement kept skin from wrinkling altogether, it would be the hottest-selling item in the world. Like many of the changes in the body after menopause, skin undergoes some inevitable deterioration with the passage of time. Lack of estrogen appears to accelerate those changes. But so do sun exposure and cigarette smoking. Indeed, the time has now come to consider deliberate sun exposure for the purpose of darkening the skin to be an exercise both in futility and folly. With or without depletion of the ozone layer, ultraviolet (UV) light not only destroys elasticity and promotes wrinkling, but it also provokes anarchy at the cellular level, leading to various forms of skin cancer. The word on the street is: deep tanning is out, Snow White is in.

6. Formication.

You're kidding!

That's for*m*ication, with an "m." Derived from the Latin word for *ant* (formica), it is a sensation that insects are crawling on the skin, experienced at least once by 15 to 20 percent of postmenopausal women. Oddly enough, it tends to occur one or two years after the last menstrual cycle. This is probably a variation on the hot flash theme, related to sudden changes in small blood vessels.

7. **Night sweats and disturbed sleep.** These symptoms are mentioned in one breath because the first often leads to

the second. Night sweats related to estrogen withdrawal are similar to hot flashes but with the added attraction of soaking nightgowns and sheets. Obviously, such an event isn't conducive to uninterrupted sleep. In addition, some women have difficulty falling asleep or staying asleep, even without the nocturnal soak.

One woman described her unique solution to this discomfiting situation: "We have to go to sleep with my husband's arm under my neck; he can *feel* me warming up and starts blowing on me. That doesn't work, of course, so I end up putting my head at the foot of the bed, right under the ceiling fan. He complains that he has a hard time finding me sometimes!" Another woman related her interrupted night life: "If I doze off, it's not long before I wake up—I have very irregular sleep patterns now. If I have a gown on, I just have to throw it off. I'm only hot at night, not during the day. I sleep with a fan (on high) blowing directly on me and I *still* wake up drenched with a hot flash—on *top* of being just plain hot. And I've always been the coldest-natured person in the world!"

What else can cause these symptoms?

Plenty, and that's why you cannot automatically assume that these events are caused by estrogen changes. Night sweats on their own may also be caused by infections or more serious illnesses, including certain malignancies. If these are occurring in the midst of hot flashes and other menopausal events, and they are relieved decisively by estrogen, then the diagnosis is straightforward. But if you have any doubt, run this problem by your physician.

Similarly, sleep disturbances may be caused by a variety of problems, especially depression. Again, if a trial of estrogen replacement brings on a dramatic improvement, the cause is probably hormonal.

8. Emotional disturbances. This is a controversial topic, one in which the medical journals seem at odds with life on the street. To quote the patient information leaflet which is provided with a commonly used estrogen preparation (Premarin®), "Sometimes women experience nervous symptoms or depression during menopause. There is no evidence that estrogens are effective for such symptoms."

In fact, for some (but certainly not all) women, estrogen replacement can have a remarkable calming effect on a stormy menopausal mood disturbance. Furthermore, the irritability, emotional swings, and general sense of being out of sorts repeats itself with striking consistency whenever the estrogen is withdrawn for a few days. The fact that some women might experience such a sensitivity to hormonal shifts should come as no surprise, unless one believes that all cases of premenstrual syndrome represent personality disturbances, and postpartum depression is a hoax—which we certainly do not.

It would be a big mistake, however, to assume that all mood disturbances surrounding menopause are strictly the product of hormonal fluctuations. Estrogen is hardly a surefire cure for everyone's irritability, anxiety, or depression. But for the right patient, estrogen can part the clouds.

It sounds like there's an awful lot of bad news that follows in the wake of this universal event in women. Is there anything else you can add to make the picture look more depressing?

Actually, we have some good news, some so-so news, and some bad news. The good news is that, while some of the structural changes (such as thinning of the vagina) are essentially universal, many women sail past menopause as if nothing much has happened. And others who are having a lot of trouble with the problems we just listed can get some impressive relief with hormone replacement therapy (HRT), even if they are not sure they want to use it on a long-term basis.

Can I apply for this "no sweat menopause" club?

Nice try. Like so many other physical characteristics, much of the response to the events of menopause is determined by genetics. Some women have a gradual decline in estrogen, for example, which tends to generate fewer symptoms than an abrupt drop or wild fluctuations in hormone levels. Others make enough estrogen in the "off site" areas (that is, away from the ovary) to limit the symptoms they experience. Also, the hypothalamus and other estrogen-responsive structures may vary in their sensitivity to hormone levels.

On the other hand, the quality of prudent self-care can make a major difference as well. Someone who is in poor condition to begin with—whether physically, emotionally, or spiritually—may find any added hormonal hassles of menopause to be intolerable. For this reason, we devote a fair amount of discussion in the next two chapters to some important preparations for this transition.

What's the so-so news you were referring to?

A reminder that many symptoms—especially flashes, flushes, and sweats—are self-limited, even without treatment.

And the bad news?

The two most potentially serious complications of estrogen withdrawal are silent until a catastrophe occurs. These are the gradual thinning of bones (osteoporosis) and the development of coronary artery disease and other complications of fatty plaque buildup within blood vessels.

What catastrophes are you talking about?

In the case of osteoporosis, the catastrophe is a fracture—

especially of the hip—from a relatively minor accident. In the case of blood vessels, it is the sudden and damaging loss of blood to part of the heart (otherwise known as a heart attack) or brain (a stroke).

These consequences are far more serious and not at all uncommon. Since a woman's risk for osteoporosis or cardio-vascular disease have a bearing on decisions regarding long-term estrogen use, these will be discussed in more detail in the chapter on Hormone Replacement Therapy.

Are there any health problems in the postmenopausal woman which aren't caused by reduced levels of estrogen?

The laundry list of postmenopausal tribulations related to reduced estrogen seems so long that it's no wonder some physicians in bygone days saw replacing this hormone as their solemn duty to the mid-life female. But in fact, while there's much to be said for hormone therapy, it can't stop the entire aging process, or every disease, or every complaint. A number of common difficulties of the peri- and postmenopausal years do not appear to be significantly affected by the ebb of estro-gen. They include the following:

1. Memory loss. Difficulty with short-term memory is so common among the aged that it has inspired comedians and writers for centuries. Paul's grandmother was mentally sharp well into her nineties; she didn't retire from choral conducting until she passed her ninetieth birthday. She summed it up with this wry lament: "I can remember music I learned as a teenager, but I can't for the life of me recall what I had for breakfast." For some this becomes a more dangerous distur-bance. They may forget food cooking on the stove or fail to take their medications. For an unfortunate few, it progresses to complete loss of intellectual capacity.

While some have suggested that estrogen might limit the aggravation of forgotten car keys or the tragedy of full-blown dementia, the majority of controlled research (so far) doesn't support such claims. It is possible, however, that concentration seems to be restored for some women when disruptive hot flashes or mood swings calm down. But don't count on estrogen to turn the mental tide if it is ebbing.

Is there anything that can be done if someone seems to be "losing it" intellectually with the passage of time?

Never assume that a person's loss of intellectual function is simply an inevitable by-product of aging. While many people do experience a relentless and horrifying progression of this problem, it is important to be sure that a treatable medical disorder isn't the underlying cause. Possibilities include hypothyroidism, a series of small strokes, low blood oxygen levels in someone with chronic lung disease, or even a slowly expanding blood clot in the skull from a seemingly minor injury. In addition, untreated depression can create a "pseudodementia" which clears with treatment.

For those with definite evidence of trouble (including specific events documented and verified by other family members), and with other medical problems ruled out, some people with mild to moderate changes have been started on the drug tacrine (Cognex®). While this may help, at least for a while, it is not the easiest medication to use. A thorough review with a primary care physician or neurologist is necessary before even considering this approach.

2. Dizziness. This word, one of the most maddeningly vague in the English language, actually encompasses a whole gamut of symptoms—a sense of dysequilibrium, a spinning sensation, faintness, or any vague feeling that "something isn't quite right" in the head. Whether the problem is impaired circulation to the inner ear (or a larger area of the brain), an unstable heart rhythm, a side effect of medication, or any of several other causes which need to be ruled out by a physician, it is very unlikely that a daily dose of estrogen will make much of a difference.

3. Heart or lung problems, with the important exception of coronary artery disease, are not related to hormones. Estrogen won't lower your blood pressure, expand your lung capacity, or improve your exercise tolerance. If you have asthma or chronic obstructive lung disease, you may need to do a number of things to improve your condition, but taking estrogen isn't one of them. However, as we will discuss in Chapter Six, women who already have coronary artery disease may still benefit from hormone replacement therapy.

4. Intestinal tract disturbances are not specifically affected by hormone withdrawal. Ulcers are driven by heredity, smoking, some medications, and certain forms of stress. At the other end of the pipeline, constipation is the most frequent intestinal complaint specifically tied to aging. The colon tends to take more and more of its sweet time to move stool, a normal tendency that can be countered by increasing fluid and fiber intake (see Chapter Three). Irritable bowel syndrome (IBS), in which the colon goes into painful spasms but without any visible signs of disease, may be provoked by stressful situations. Estrogen may indirectly reduce this annoying problem because it can improve the woman's overall sense of well-being, thereby reducing stress.

5. Aches and pains in the joints, muscles, and ligaments. As noted, we will look at osteoporosis, which estrogen helps prevent, in Chapter Six. But estrogen does not stop arthritis, whether arising from years of wear and tear on the weight-bearing joints or more widespread immune disorders such as rheumatoid arthritis. And it will not prevent muscle strain (especially in the neck and low back), bursitis, or other common musculoskeletal problems.

6. Decline in kidney function. While estrogen withdrawal causes atrophy of the lower end of the urinary tract, the kidneys are not specifically affected. However, they do undergo a gradual loss over time in their efficiency as the body's filter system. This is reflected in the results of a test called the serum creatinine, which almost invariably creeps upward slightly with age. In the post-seventy-five set, or at any age in which known kidney disease has been discovered, medication doses may have to be adjusted to compensate for this inevitable change in kidney function.

7. Anxiety and depression.

I thought you said that estrogen would calm emotional storms after menopause?

It will—in some people. But many women who develop these very common mood disturbances during and after the mid-life years need much more than estrogen. We will take a longer look at these issues in Chapter Five.

*   *   *

This laundry list isn't any more encouraging than your other one. What can be done to head off some of these other problems?

A detailed look at the entire gamut of medical problems that may crop up during the menopausal years is beyond the scope of this book (and might be too depressing). But there are several important health issues which are common, preventable, and often detectable by screening tests before they set off full-blown symptoms. We are therefore going to press on in the next chapter with a look at some basic "preventive maintenance" measures which contribute to an optimal physical condition and fewer repair bills. And in Chapter Seven we will tour the screening tests which can help uncover the most common troublemakers before they progress too far. Stay with us.

Chapter Three

How Do I Get Ready?
Part I: Physical Preparations

The book of Genesis describes the seductive promises used in the temptation of the first man and woman: if they would assert their own will and disobey God, they would (1) be like God and (2) never die. This, of course, was the penultimate lie, because the resulting fallen creation very resoundingly declares (1) how very ungodlike we are and (2) the inevitability of our death.

In our youthfulness, it is difficult to grasp the enormity of what Christ did at the cross to reverse this bleak situation because we feel so powerfully alive. But as we approach our middle years, the cumulative effects of aging begin to drive home the truth we have been ignoring for decades: this body will not last forever. During these middle years, we begin to confront the stuff of which our faith is made. We truly learn, as never before, that our citizenship is not in this present body. "Who we are" resides not in these frail vessels, but in a soul which has been redeemed *away from* a time-limited physical body.

So do we just drop out of life, sit around in the lotus position and meditate while waiting to leave this temporary residence? Hardly! The apostle Paul, while writing from prison, cheerfully explained his outlook: "I eagerly expect and hope that I will in no way be ashamed, but will have sufficient courage so that now as always Christ will be exalted in my body" (Phil 1:20). Paul certainly had the right idea: that his mind and body were valuable *tools*, means to an end. And his goal was to serve God for as long as he could draw breath. If we could get a tight grip on this concept, we would be properly motivated to take excellent care of our bodies without worshiping them as if they were going to last forever.

It's a shame that so many years of abuse may have to accumulate before we get the idea that our bodies are a finite resource! Suddenly the ten pounds we could drop in two weeks at age twenty-five (by simply cutting out the midnight ice cream) now seem resistant to months of self-discipline and exercise. We sheepishly wait for the aisle to clear at the supermarket before reaching for our first box of hair coloring. A comfortable flannel nightgown has long since replaced the sexy stuff. And you *know* you're finally starting to face your own mortality when you wake up one morning, look groggily into the mirror and wonder, for the first time, how much a face-lift costs.

The bad news is that good health does not happen accidentally. If you're in your middle years (and why would you be reading this if you weren't?) you hopefully have discovered that by now. The really *good* news is that it doesn't take a lot of money or time to increase dramatically your chances for enjoying a long and robust life in a healthy body. Long-term discipline brings long-term fitness, not a sudden and short-lived New Year's resolution that involves killing yourself at a gym two hours a day, five days a week!

After trying one entrepreneurial "this-one's-going-to-make-us-rich" scheme after another (with no lasting results), Teri's dad finally settled down, at the age of forty-five, to a steady job that began with a modest salary. For the next twenty years, he faithfully invested a small percentage of every paycheck. When he retired, he had accumulated a small fortune from his steady, conservative investments—far more than he would have with any of his incredible schemes, and with *far* less stress to his long-suffering wife!

Physical, mental, and emotional/spiritual "wealth" is much the same: it is the day-to-day *small but steady* investment that pays off big dividends eventually. Why waste the next ten years of your life forever *planning* the major changes you're going to make in your life, when you can begin *today* with a modest investment plan that will pay off big? Your menopause years are not going to wait while you express eternal best intentions to get it all together, just as the first labor pain doesn't wait for the last class to end. Begin today getting prepared for the rest of your life.

After reading through all of the ravages of age and declining estrogen levels that you detailed in the last chapter, I wonder if it's really worth trying to "fight city hall." How can I possibly prepare myself for all of these impending disasters?

Sorry, we didn't mean to make things sound so bleak. Remember that the changes your body will experience do not all lead to discomfort and disease. More importantly, it is amazing how many medical problems can be circumvented by making some very basic lifestyle decisions and sticking to them. We present here the concept of a **"Basic Maintenance Checklist"**—a few key areas which may sound like very familiar refrains because they affect so many areas of physical health.

Is this going to be another one of those "Lose weight/Exercise/Don't smoke/Mind your mother" speeches, like my doctor gives me in fifteen seconds as he's rushing out the exam room door?

Well, it'll last more than fifteen seconds. And we'll try not to make it too glib, because changing long-standing habits is so much easier said than done (as witnessed by the shelves full of books at the library or bookstore on most of these subjects). *But we cannot emphasize enough how important the following items can be to your overall well-being during the coming decades.* Our desire here is to motivate you to take these seriously, to work on them, and to stay with them.

All right, so what's on your famous Basic Maintenance Checklist?

So glad you asked. The list is as follows:

1. Attain and maintain an appropriate weight.
2. Use low fat and high fiber fuel.
3. Move your muscles.
4. Deal with your lipids if they're too high.
5. Deal with your blood pressure if it's elevated.
6. Get smoke out of your life.
7. Adjust your alcohol intake.
8. Wear your seatbelt.
9. Keep your sex life a "closed system."

Good night, Irene! You do sound like my mother, except you forgot to say "Brush your teeth" and "Put on your mittens." Do I really have to wade through this?

Not if you've got all of these areas figured out and optimized. Otherwise, humor us by taking another brief look at these topics.

Why?

Because if everyone actually *followed* all of these well-supported recommendations (we didn't just make them up) successfully and consistently throughout life, at least half of the almost trillion dollar annual health care bill in our country would be eliminated. Many people would spare themselves and their families untold physical pain, mental anguish, and economic hardship, and they would live much longer. Individual well-being and energy, not to mention national productivity levels, would markedly improve. Hopefully one of these benefits might appeal to you.

OK, OK. You can dismount the soapbox and fire when ready.

1. Attain and maintain an appropriate weight.

Why do you have to put weight at the top of the list?

Mainly because some of the other problem areas—particularly blood pressure and lipids—have a way of improving when one's weight is where it belongs.

Why do you say "appropriate" rather than "ideal" weight?

Because the word "ideal" sounds like something unattainable, the property of some sleek model on a magazine cover. The pursuit of that image drives many women to plunge into unhealthy crash diets, or discourages them so much whenever they check the mirror that they never get started. You do not have to be shaped like someone in the *Sports Illustrated* swimsuit edition to be healthy and attractive.

The word *appropriate* also indicates that, while excessive weight is the most common nutritional problem in our country, one can also reach a point of diminishing returns while feverishly driving the scale past the low one hundreds.

So there is no medical support for the famous bumper sticker wisdom, "You can't be too rich or too thin"?

You certainly *can* be too thin. Having an extremely low weight does not contribute to longevity; it may stop menses prematurely, contribute to osteoporosis (thinning of bone), and adversely affect skin and hair, among other problems. An obsessive need to be a little thinner, no matter what you weigh, may represent a significant problem of self-image for which professional help (both psychological and dietary) should be sought. But as we move through our forties and beyond, the biggest nutritional problem in Western cultures is definitely excess poundage.

I've wondered if there was something wrong with me over the years, because I seem to gain weight continually without changing my diet or activity patterns. Is that unusual?

Not at all. Primary care doctors hear this lament every day. Obviously, your body doesn't suction weight out of thin air, and rarely does a medical disorder prove to be the cause of this amazing phenomenon. The only relatively common exception is fluid retention, which can be brought on by disorders of heart, kidney, and thyroid function, not to mention the cyclic fluid shifts that many women experience. Typically this manifests as significant and sudden changes in weight, in either direction, which are virtually impossible with fat.

Why do you say that rapid changes in weight aren't related to fat?

Fat metabolism is an engineering marvel, an automatic mechanism which efficiently deals with fluctuations in food supply by stashing away extra energy when we take in more food than we need, and then retrieving it when we consume less food than will meet our energy needs. As it turns out, each pound of fat represents about thirty-five hundred calories of fuel storage. This means that the most rapid fat loss one could possibly generate—with no food intake whatsoever and moderate levels of activity—would be in the range of eight to twelve ounces per day. Such an unhealthy and miserable scenario would (at best) trim three to five pounds per week. When the tabloids proclaim the next wonder diet that sheds ten pounds in five days, remember that the vast majority of that weight reduction comes from a transient diuresis (a quick loss of fluid via the kidneys) that occurs universally when calories out exceed calories in.

So if there's no magic weight loss, why does my weight seem to go up as if by magic?

Because nearly every adult becomes more fuel efficient as the years pass. What kept your body going twenty years ago is more than it needs today. Since few of us automatically lose our hunger pangs and gastronomic tastes as the years pass, the net effect is a gradual accumulation of the proverbial "spare tire."

Not only does biology promote this weight gain, but almost every convenience and advance of modern life appears destined to add to our girth. We ride instead of walk, use elevators instead of stairs, and jam our calendars so full of commitments that an hour of deliberate exercise represents a major sacrifice. To top it off, we have a huge supply of calories readily available from the fast food restaurant and the corner grocery store. Virtually every social gathering, project, entertainment, and mood shift is an occasion to eat. In fact, hunger is rarely the event that triggers food-seeking behavior. Given this stacked deck, it's a wonder that everyone isn't obese.

Why is this process so hard to reverse, especially in women? So often I hear about men who simply decide to skip dessert and cut back on fats, and their weight sinks like a stone.

This is a reality of metabolism which probably conferred some survival value in bygone generations. Think about it: the current abundance of food among developed countries is unprecedented in the history of the world. When food supplies are scarce, guess who lives the longest: those who burn up their fat stores the slowest. (Paul routinely congratulates his patients who complain about difficult weight loss, reminding them that they are the best equipped for a famine. They are usually not amused.)

Women who lose a great deal of weight usually stop their normal menstrual cycles, a common medical issue among extremely lean female athletes. They are not fertile, and thus not capable of perpetuating the human race. Therefore, most likely by design, females do not typically shed weight as readily as their male counterparts. Furthermore, the increased fuel efficiency later in life probably has assisted survival over the centuries. If the elderly burned calories as quickly as two-year-olds, few would have lived to a "ripe old age" before this century.

All of this theory is interesting, but how does it help me at this point in time?

We only mention it as a reminder that you're not unique, sick, or victimized if you are having a hard time losing weight. And we also mention it to introduce the *very* important concept that weight management is not some quick fix—a few weeks of suffering followed by "business as usual"—but a lifelong process.

So you're not big on diet pills?

Nor on magical food supplements, or "diets" in general. To say "I'm on a diet" is similar to saying "I'm serving a prison sentence for my crimes." The diet and the prison sentence are both miserable experiences, from which parole or escape looks better with each passing week. Diet pills are nothing but various forms of "uppers" (ranging from common decongestants to full-blown amphetamines), and the miracle supplements (usually hocked in the comic section of the Sunday paper, where they belong) which "melt away fat in your sleep" or allow you to "eat anything you want and still lose weight" are bogus.

I do plan to steer clear of those bozos. But what about outfits such as Jenny Craig or Nutri-System?

These plans are legitimate and will work, but they also consume some bucks, since you typically buy your food as well as attend classes at the franchise office. For the person who doesn't want to spend a lot of time preparing food, having everything done for you can be very helpful. But you can't live on the pre-packaged food forever, and it is extremely important to follow through with the full maintenance course. One of the worst (but all too common) traps for the overweight is the "rhythm method of girth control"—the yo-yo pattern of weight loss and gain caused by drifting in and out of various diet plans. After a few of these adventures, the body actually becomes less cooperative with your goals.

What about all of those diet plans I see at the bookstore? Could I just follow one of those?

Certainly, provided that you're not dealing with nutritional information from another planet. Some of the most popular diet books in recent decades have been amazingly wrong-headed, nearsighted, or overtly ridiculous. One popular author, for example, not long ago suggested that carbohydrates caused weight gain, and that eating nothing but "high protein" foods (i.e., meats) would tip the scale downward. Of course, these foods tend to have higher fat and cholesterol content, and so these dieters unknowingly were driving up their risk of coronary artery disease, whether or not they lost any weight. Another bizarre notion claims that one should combine only certain types of foods at any given meal or dire consequences will ensue. How the human race managed to survive before the discovery of these essential combinations is, of course, unexplained.

A good book on nutrition and weight loss stresses basic *patterns* of eating rather than nit-picking about particular foods and supplements, and also deals with some of the healthy *attitudes* about food that lead to better choices. One of our favorites for several years has been *Jane Brody's Nutrition Book* and its companion volume, *Jane Brody's Good Food Book*. A nutrition columnist for the *New York Times*, Ms. Brody has done her homework and written in an interesting and informative style about all facets of the food we consume. Her section on weight loss is excellent and highly recommended. Another outstanding resource is *Love Hunger* by a team of authors from the Minirth-Meier Clinics. This book combines nutritional information with a detailed assessment of forces that drive excessive eating and strategies to deal with them.

So what do you consider the key ingredients in a successful approach to this problem?

Thought you'd never ask. All of these, by the way, are not absolutely necessary for progress to be made. But those who obtain the best results—both short and, most importantly, long-term—seem to adopt the majority of these concepts.

1. Eliminate the phrase "I'm on a diet" from your speech

and your behavior. You should adopt new eating patterns for the long haul—in fact, plan on them lasting for the rest of your life. If you can barely tolerate the way you are eating to lose weight, your losses are bound to be temporary.

2. Plan for a long, slow reduction in weight. Consuming one thousand calories less per day than you use will yield an average of two pounds off per week, which is a very respectable rate (but very possibly difficult to sustain). A more leisurely five hundred calorie discrepancy leads to a slower loss of one pound per week. This may not sound like much, but it's a whopping fifty pounds over a year of consistency. Remember: quick losses almost always are transient and are quickly regained in a destructive yo-yo pattern.

3. Fall in love with low fat foods. If you can't fall in love with them, figure out ways to like them. As we will point out in the next section of the Basic Maintenance Checklist, a variety of health problems improve when fatty foods are banished from one's body.

What do you mean by low fat foods?

For the most part, these are foods derived from vegetables, fruits, and grains. Most of the fat at our table comes from animal sources (meats, eggs, dairy products) and oils, which are derived from a variety of plants. Total elimination of animal products is unnecessary, but they need to be scaled way down and chosen wisely. There's a world of difference between a piece of nicely seasoned skinless baked chicken and a hunk of the same bird deep fried in calorie-drenched oil. We will not bore you here with a laundry list of advisable vs. bad news foods, but the books we have mentioned provide this information.

4. Eat only when the hypothalamus asks for food—in other words, when you're feeling some hunger. As mentioned earlier, we eat for every reason in the world except actual hunger pangs. A detailed examination of the needs that food can

meet—comfort, control, tranquilization, a break, and so on—and alternative methods of meeting those needs is contained in *Love Hunger*.

Some weight loss plans have advocated the "single plate/single setting" approach to help distinguish true hunger from random eating. This involves choosing a single distinctive (but not very large) plate and a particular location (usually the kitchen or dining room table), and deciding that, when at home, one will eat only from the one plate at the one setting. While eating, nothing else is to be done: no reading, watching TV, working on projects, etc. So if you get the urge for a bag of microwave popcorn, go right ahead—but you have to sit and eat it, with nothing else going on, from the special plate at the single setting.

This behavior modification technique is meant to separate food from all of the other irrelevant activities which accompany it, and in the process make eating a boring process of quelling hunger. But it also violates the "live with this forever" rule, and it is destined to be scrapped sooner or later—undoubtedly with a ceremonial smashing of the special plate.

5. On the other hand, don't skip meals.

You mean all of that propaganda from Health Ed. about breakfast being such an important meal is true?

Afraid so. The common practice of charging off to work or school with a cup of coffee, grabbing a snack for lunch, and then sitting down to dinner as the main meal of the day doesn't make sense. Meals should correlate with activity levels, not socialization. If food has been left out of a busy schedule, a lot of hunger combined with the need to relax may result in a feeding frenzy followed by doing nothing. This pattern may suit the lifestyle of a boa constrictor, but not a healthy human being.

Also, don't assume that you have to wait for traditional mealtimes to eat. These are social conventions, not universal laws. Some people do much better eating frequent small amounts of food rather than two or three big chomp sessions driven by ravenous hunger. In fact, one study on weight reduction successfully utilized a virtual "grazing" program of low-fat foods eaten—get this—seventeen times per day.

6. Take your time at the table. The feedback loop from intestine to bloodstream to brain that says "I'm not hungry any more" doesn't close any faster when food is inhaled than when it is savored in smaller amounts. For many of us, the satisfaction of eating is related to the duration of the meal, not necessarily the amount. If, in a given time frame, a smaller amount of food is eaten, fewer calories will need to be disposed of.

7. Work some accountability into your plan. Remember that we tend to practice the piano more fervently as the day of the weekly lesson approaches. Knowing that someone is paying attention and following your progress can engage an important mental force: the intense and universal desire not to look like an idiot.

This is one reason why groups such as Weight Watchers and TOPS (Take Off Pounds Sensibly) are a worthwhile and successful use of time and (a little) money. Their approaches properly stress the long haul, their advice is mainstream and sensible, and their weekly "weigh-in" provokes compliance that internal motivaters rarely can duplicate.

8. Start moving your muscles. We will get into this as the third item on the Basic Maintenance Checklist, but half an hour of moderate exercise (such as a brisk walk) is an important adjunct to your efforts.

Can I lose weight by eating the same as always but doing more exercise?

Many people have an unrealistic notion of the number of calories they will burn during exercise, and then they complain when increasing activity doesn't lead to dramatic weight loss. If exercise is to be your primary mode of losing weight, plan on spending most of your day doing it. For example, without altering food intake, the average adult would need to walk about thirty-five miles to lose one pound of fat. That's five miles per day to make a modest one pound dent every week.

So what's the point of exercising?

There are lots of points, as we'll see momentarily. But while expending some (if not massive) calories, exercise improves one's overall sense of energy and well-being, which in turn leads to more activity throughout the day. Exercise also tends to curb the appetite. And the memory of the huffing and puffing may inspire some better decisions later. ("If I worked my fanny off on the stair-stepper this morning, I sure don't want to undo it by eating this cheesecake.")

9. Check the scale only once or twice per week. The important issue is the overall trend of weight, not day-to-day fluctuations. Nothing is so frustrating as to struggle with new eating habits for a few days and then find out that weight went *up*. Such a disheartening paradox may occur with fluid shifts during the course of a month and may not truly reflect the progress you have made.

So if I abide by the Nine Commandments above, I'll lose weight without any problem, right?

If losing weight were a piece of cake (pardon the figure of speech), obesity would not be such a major national health problem, and there wouldn't be so many diet books and programs on the market. Making sensible changes, and staying with them for months and years, is far easier said than done. The basic perspectives listed so far (more like the Nine Suggestions) are important, but physical, emotional, and social factors obviously enter the equation as well.

You got that right. I have got a major problem at home because I prepare the meals for the whole family. How can I stay on my di—I mean, new eating habits— when I have to deal with everyone else's food as well? I feel like an alcoholic who's on the wagon but living in a saloon.

If your food choices are going to be successful, they shouldn't be radically different from what everyone else at home is eating. In fact, the rest of the family ought to be in the low-fat zone as well. (You need to be careful about "sampling" the food several times during preparation, however, because quantity is obviously important.) And if everyone puts up a fuss because you're making healthy changes (serving broiled chicken and fish instead of burgers and dogs, for example), tell them it's because you care about their health. If they don't like what you prepare, they can fend for themselves.

I find I can do well for a while, and then I completely blow it on some occasion. Doesn't that negate all of the good decisions I've made?

Absolutely not, unless by "blowing it" you mean a huge binge (whole packages of cookies, quarts of ice cream, entire bags of chips, etc.). Remember that backsliding for a few hours or a day can only alter your fat storage by a few ounces at the very most. It is the ongoing *pattern* of eating that matters. Please note: if getting off track for you involves bingeing, the kind of mass consumption mentioned above, it is extremely important that you begin counseling. The issues involved with your eating go far beyond the basic arithmetic of calories.

The mention of counseling brings us to one final ingredient (to round things out to an even Ten Suggestions):

10. If you absolutely do not see progress after an honest effort over a reasonable amount of time (say three months), get some help from a registered dietitian. A diary detailing a few days of *everything* eaten during that time should be brought along. Don't forget that everyone stores and burns fuel at different rates, and you may have been dealt an unfavorable biological hand. Rather than pining about it, find out what the realities are for you. The dietitian may find a few big wads of unsuspected calories hiding in your food choices. Remember: you always get more from an expert when you have struggled with the problem on your own for a while.

Let's move on now to the second point on our Basic Maintenance Checklist.

2. Use Low Fat / High Fiber Fuel.

I thought you just went over this.

We did bring it up in the last section, but our admonition now doesn't merely apply to those who need to shed weight. It is possible, if the quantities are right, to maintain a very reasonable weight while consuming fuel with the wrong blend: too much fat, too much simple carbohydrate (the various sugars), too little complex carbohydrate, too little fiber.

I've been hearing so much about fiber over the past few years that you'd think it was the greatest thing since sliced bread. What exactly is fiber, and why all the hype?

The generic term *fiber* actually refers to a variety of substances derived from fruits, vegetables, and grains. *Soluble* fiber includes pectin and oat bran, which contribute to healthy hearts by helping escort cholesterol out of the body. *Insoluble* fiber is found on the outside husks of rice, wheat, and vegetable skins, and passes through the intestinal tract virtually without being digested.

In the late 1970s Dr. Dennis Burkitt—a deeply committed Christian, by the way—published some important observations after serving as a medical missionary in Africa for twenty years. He noted among his patients a virtual absence of diseases so common in the Western world: appendicitis, diverticulitis, cancer of the colon, gallstones, even hemorrhoids. He also found that they consumed far greater amounts of dietary fiber in the form of vegetables, fruits, and unrefined grains, and they usually passed two or more large, soft stools every day.

This is appetizing. What's the point?

Burkitt proposed that the softening and bulking effect of the undigested fiber increases the speed with which food travels through the intestines and makes the food-moving job of the intestinal muscles much easier. This would in turn limit the contact of carcinogens (cancer-provoking agents) with the inner surface of the colon; reduce the pressure and squeezing which contributes to formation of diverticuli (literally, "little diversions," the small outpouchings from the colon that can become infected, or even perforate); decrease the likelihood that a hard little wad of stool will get stuck in the appendix, leading to appendicitis; and reduce absorption of cholesterol, which not only contributes to choked arteries but forms most gallstones. Obviously, if you pass one or more soft stools a day, constipation and straining (which help form hemorrhoids) aren't a problem, either.

I've heard that there might be a connection between fat in the diet and breast cancer. Is that true?

The literature is not conclusive on this issue. In fact, one purpose of the massive Women's Health Initiative mentioned in Chapter One is to clarify this question. But a reduced risk of breast cancer may indeed prove to be a benefit of low fat fuel.

Any other advantages, while we're on the subject?

Reduction in blood lipid levels, which affects the risk of coronary artery disease, usually accompanies the shift to less fat and more fiber. (We'll discuss this extremely important health problem a bit later.) Another benefit of this emphasis, for those of us who love eating in general, is that we can consume larger quantities without increasing the calorie load. Carbohydrates contain four calories per gram, while fats contain nine. And fruits and vegetables contain more bites and bulk than fatty foods, so we can feel full and satisfied while reducing our overall fuel consumption.

Do you have any specific suggestions on shifting to low-fat and high-fiber fuel consumption?

Here are two pearls of wisdom which will guarantee compliance:
1. "If it had a face, don't eat it."
2. "If it tastes good, spit it out."
But seriously, there are a few more realistic general guidelines.

1. Current nutritional wisdom calls for fat to contribute less than 30 percent of your total calorie intake per day. (Most Americans consume 40 percent or more of their fuel as fat.) Likewise, complex carbohydrates should account for more than 50 percent of the calorie total. Since most of us don't walk around with calorie computers strapped to our belts, this boils down to some basic concepts:

a. Instead of fatty meats and fried foods, substitute fish, skinless chicken and turkey, and lean meats. And think in terms of limiting "high protein" foods (which were all the rage a decade ago), such as meat, poultry, and eggs to three to six ounces per day.

b. Eliminate full-fat dairy products (such as whole milk and gourmet ice cream) in favor of low-fat alternative. Remember that nonfat or 1 percent milk is an excellent source of protein and calcium without a high fat content. In nonfat milk 10 percent of the calories are fat (so it's not *completely* nonfat), while in 1 percent milk the fat ratio is 16 percent. But get this: in 2 percent milk fat calories rise to 25 percent, and in whole milk to 50 percent! The news is worse for most cheeses, which soar into the 70 to 90 percent fat zone.

c. Limit daily cholesterol to 300 mg. per day. Better yet, limit it to 150 mg. per day. (Keep in mind that one egg yolk contains 250 mg.)

d. Eat five or more half-cup servings of vegetables and fruits, and six or more servings of bread, cereals, or legumes per day.

e. Remember to shun the infamous saturated fats in favor of those of the polyunsaturated and monounsaturated persuasion.

I've heard these terms for years and haven't a clue what they mean. What's the difference?

Without getting into organic chemistry, let's just say that saturated fats are the most likely to contribute to plugged arteries. These are abundant in whole milk products, palm and coconut oils, and hydrogenated oils and shortenings. Polyunsaturated fats, such as are found in vegetable oils, help lower cholesterol levels. Monounsaturated fats, found in olive oil, are considered the healthiest of the lot. But remember that these all are equally dense in calories, saturated or not.

2. Learn to read nutritional information labels on food products you buy. You can get a quick grip on the percentages of fat by multiplying the number of grams of fat in a serving by nine, which will give you the number of fat calories per serving. Divide that by the total number of calories per serving, multiply by one hundred, and you'll get the percentage of fat in the food. If it's over 30 percent, leave it on the shelf.

3. Try to eat at least twenty-five grams of crude fiber per day. Gravitate toward whole grain breads and cereals, and check the packages for quantities. (Fiber One® cereal, for example, has a hefty twenty-one grams per ounce.) Peas, beans (not string), blackberries, and raspberries have particularly high fiber levels. But don't count on green salads to provide much fiber—unless they have a lot of other ingredients besides lettuce, which carries a bare .8 gm per cup. You may want to consider adding wheat bran (more than 40 percent fiber) or fiber supplements such as Metamucil® or Citrucel® to your daily routine.

I'm afraid if I load up with all this fiber, I'm going to spend my whole life in the bathroom.

If you're not used to going every day, get used to it. Believe it or not, two or three times per day is OK, as long as the stools are formed. In fact, it would be wise to increase fluid intake if your fiber input has gone up, in order to prevent constipation.

4. Here's a tough one for some: minimize the overtly sweet foods. Watch out especially for soft drinks, which contain the equivalent of more than ten teaspoons of sugar per can. While sugar is certainly not the root of all evil, as has been claimed by some over the years, it is a relatively dense calorie source without anything else to offer.

3. Move your muscles.

I'm on my feet and on the go all day long. Are you saying I need to be spending more time in my day doing some sort of sweaty workout?

Congratulations—in one question you've hit on most of the obstacles which interfere with one of the simplest but most important factors of health maintenance. The daily agenda is crammed so full that, for many of us, a half hour spent exercising seems like a major sacrifice. Timing can be a hassle, especially if there's a full-time job to contend with. Who wants to get up at the crack of dawn, or else try to get all cranked up doing exercise when it would be nicer just to relax after an intense day at work? And who can keep up with those sleek trainers on the video or at the health club without feeling totally wiped out?

You took the words right out of my mouth.

Well, we've got good news and bad news. The bad news is that without some sort of deliberate, daily muscle motion you will be treading the "broad road that leads to destruction." The sedentary lifestyle may be the path of least resistance, but it is not without costs. The good news is that exercise does not need to be such a big production in order to gain some major benefits.

What might those be?

Decreased risk of obesity, heart disease, high blood pressure, and diabetes; stronger bones; less stiffness, aches, and pains; and a longer life. Not to mention increased stamina, mental alertness, and an overall improved sense of well-being.

Come on, nothing is that all-encompassing in its effects.

Actually, a large scale study (involving more than 13,000 subjects) conducted by the Institute for Aerobics Research in Dallas, Texas showed that even a very modest level of exercise reduced the overall death rate (not just limited to heart disease), compared with those who were sedentary.

Paul has noted that, with the passage of time, it becomes increasingly apparent in the exam room when someone has been a consistent exerciser. It may not be so obvious among those in their twenties and thirties, but as the years motor past the late forties, the more physically fit begin to stand out as the "low maintenance" patients. They look better, feel better, have fewer complaints, and fewer office visits.

Let's zero in on that "very modest" level of exercise you mentioned. How much are we talking about?

A half-hour walk, four times per week.

That's it?

That's it: a very simple target for most people. No special equipment, no health club, no expenses, no huge strain on the body, not much of a time commitment.

Any precautions?

A few. First, run this by your physician. Chances are he or she will heartily approve of your plans, since very few health problems improve with inactivity. But problems such an unstable heart condition, significant arthritis or other orthopedic issues, diabetes, or significant obesity, to name a few, may need some prior clearance.

The surface should be flat. Traversing up and down rolling

hills can be far more taxing on heart, bones, and joints. Surroundings should be safe and pleasant. Inclement weather, the heat of the day, the dead of night, and any generally hazardous conditions (such as traffic) would be best avoided. Many people do their walking exercise in large shopping malls, where the climate is controlled and the chances of a mugging or a canine encounter are definitely reduced. Of course, stopping to window shop or grab a fast food snack can defeat the whole purpose of being there, so a little self-control is necessary.

If you live in an area with character-building climate, a treadmill can be an excellent use of a few hundred dollars (or less). With this device you can work out whenever you want, but make sure it's in a place that's "user friendly." Nothing is less enticing than trekking out to a cluttered, cold, smelly garage for a wonderful half hour of exercise.

Finally, make sure you stretch your calves and hamstrings for a few minutes at the outset.

Once you have completed a few sessions, begin to measure your distance. Try to increase your speed gradually until you cover two miles in the half hour. This may be relatively easy, or it may take you weeks, depending on your initial conditioning level.

How do I prevent getting bored with this, week in and week out?

Bring someone with you—spouse, kids, neighbor, dog, whatever—for company and conversation. (We have a lot of "debriefing" and other pleasant discussions during our own walks.) Vary your route so you don't look at the same scenery every time. Spend time thinking and praying about the people you care for. Buy a portable cassette recorder and listen to some tapes; a half hour goes by very quickly when you're engrossed in a great message or a book on cassette.

(Many public libraries have sizable collections of recorded books.)

What if I don't want to walk as my form of exercise?

Excellent question. We brought up the walk first because it is so simple. But the primary object is to increase heart rate and oxygen consumption for a sustained period of time, in what is called aerobic exercise. This can take many forms, most of which are more vigorous than walking: jogging, swimming, cycling, cross-country skiing, and aerobic dancing, as well as the many popular workouts on video. If you are already actively pursuing one of these activities, you don't necessarily need to downgrade as you get older. But any quantum leap in aerobic exercise should be preceded by a discussion with your physician, and possibly a treadmill (stress test) to be sure that your heart is up to the task.

You gave a specific time and distance goal for walking. What about similar goals for the other activities?

No matter what form of aerobic activity you undertake, two principles are extremely important. First, it is far better to do a little bit every day than to punctuate a sedentary existence with sudden bouts of heavy exertion. The first approach protects you against the development of coronary artery disease, but the second may actually provoke a heart attack in someone whose blood vessels are already compromised.

Second, it is important to increase the duration and vigor of exertion gradually over several weeks, rather than to try going "zero to sixty" in the first few days. Some of the most useful guidelines for these increments of exercise have been published in the books of Kenneth Cooper, M.D., one of the first physicians to research and disseminate the benefits of aerobics. *Aerobics for Women* and *The Aerobics Program for Total*

Well Being are classics in this field and should be available at the public library if not at your local bookstore. These volumes contain age-specific charts for a variety of activities, providing detailed, step-by-step guidelines for conditioning over several weeks.

Just as we discussed with eating, there are bound to be setbacks and lapses with any behavior change. In the case of exercise, these may cause a regression in conditioning, such that a lower level of exertion will have to serve as the point of re-entry. But by no means give up. In fact, with consistent activity over a period of weeks, most people develop a positive addiction to the sense of well-being that exercise provides. We hope you will have this experience and your muscle motion will develop into a long-standing habit.

4. Deal with your lipids if they're too high.

And by lipids you mean . . .

Total cholesterol, HDL, LDL, and triglycerides.

Could we define a few terms?

Of course. First of all, the term *lipids* refers to all of the circulating molecules which are derived from, or participate in the production of, fatty tissue. The most important of these, for our discussion, are the various forms of cholesterol and triglycerides.

I've been hearing a lot about cholesterol lately, and none of it sounds very good.

Actually, cholesterol is an important compound, present in nearly all cells, and the foundation for several important hormones and other substances. We always have (and need) *some* of it in circulation, whether synthsesized internally or absorbed from food. And as you probably have heard, this famous molecule is abundant in cheese, eggs, fried foods, red meat, shellfish....

...and all the other foods that taste good?

Right. As might be expected, cholesterol tends to be more abundant in foods derived from animals. That's why we have so much more trouble with it in well-developed, affluent cultures, which have an abundance of meat and dairy products, as opposed to people in third world nations, who have very few animal products in their diet.

So what kind of trouble does cholesterol cause?

When it is overly concentrated in the bloodstream as it travels to its various destinations, cholesterol can contribute to the formation of fatty plaques inside of blood vessels. These plaques can become thick and dense enough to block the flow of blood, or they create ragged surfaces which can attract platelets. Platelets are cleverly designed "mini cells" which function as clot-starters, circulating through blood vessels, seeking holes or tears to plug. They attach to any rough surfaces they find, and then attract various proteins (called clotting factors) which build a formal clot. As a result, blood vessels can be clogged gradually by what physicians call atherosclerotic plaque ("athero" = "fatty" and "sclero-" = "hardened"), or suddenly by a blood clot.

What happens when blood vessels become clogged?

The biblical declaration that "the life is in the blood" (Lev 17:11, 14 and others) is absolutely true. Every cell in the body needs a steady supply of oxygen, which is carried and delivered by red cells. Tissues become unhappy when the need for oxygen outstrips the supply, and they usually complain by generating pain. The leg muscles, for example, may respond to a short walk with a terrible aching (called "claudication"), and then quiet down with rest. The heart muscle may do likewise with exercise or excitement (or sometimes spontaneously), producing a squeezing chest discomfort known as angina.

If the blood supply to any tissue is cut off suddenly by a clot, the results can be disastrous (unless the flow is restored very quickly) because that tissue will die. An unresolved clot in the leg will lead to an amputation. If any of the coronary arteries are blocked, the dying heart muscle may generate dangerous unstable rhythms which can cause sudden death. And when any part of the brain loses its vital blood supply, the results are so immediately evident that the term *stroke* (as in lightning) is applied to this event.

The disability, suffering, and expense generated by choked and clogged blood vessels are incalculable. In fact, they represent the leading direct cause of death every year. Because these problems are so common and so devastating, looking out for the well-being of your arteries—*well before there are any signs or symptoms*—is extremely important.

And the higher the cholesterol level in the bloodstream, the more the arteries become clogged, right?

Generally speaking, yes. There are always exceptions to the rule and variations on the theme. But the higher your cholesterol concentration climbs past two hundred (measured as milligrams of cholesterol per one hundred cubic centimeters of blood, for you compulsive chemistry fans), and the longer it stays there, the greater the odds that the fatty plaque is quietly accumulating in your blood vessels.

How far above 200 is considered significant?

Generally, total cholesterol levels up to 240 are considered "mild to moderate," while those over 240 pose a significant risk. However, lower levels can be worrisome in the presence of other risk factors (especially smoking, high blood pressure, and diabetes) or an unfavorable balance of HDL and LDL.

That's your second reference to HDL and LDL. I'm not in the mood for a biochemistry lecture, but why are these initials important?

Since cholesterol is a fatty substance, and blood is water based, cholesterol would form oily clumps if it were left to circulate on its own. In order to disperse evenly throughout the bloodstream, cholesterol molecules are attached to carriers called lipoproteins, which literally serve as their escorts. But to complicate matters, there are a variety of lipoproteins, with seemingly different agendas. The two most famous types are the LDL (or *low density lipoprotein*) and HDL (*high density lipoprotein*). LDL seems to allow cholesterol to plaster itself to the inner walls of blood vessels, while HDL may "scavenge" cholesterol and reduce plaque.

As an illustration, imagine that you could ride in your car only if it were loaded on a flatbed truck. Think of your car as a cholesterol molecule, the truck as a lipoprotein molecule, and the highway as an artery. The drivers of LDL flatbeds are disorderly and reckless, dumping cars all over the road and blocking the highways, while HDL drivers are "environmentally minded," not only carrying their own cargo but picking up some of the other wrecks as well.

For lack of more erudite language, we can unofficially dub cholesterol attached to LDL as "bad" and that carried by HDL as "good." The bottom line is that LDL (bad) cholesterol should be less than 130 (in the same units). Levels up to 160 are considered to pose a mild to moderate risk, while those over 190 are significant enough to warrant active intervention.

HDL ideally should be higher than 45, and levels over 60 are considered "protective" of the heart's blood supply. Some laboratories divide the total cholesterol by the HDL to yield a "coronary risk ratio." Since ideally the total cholesterol should be as low as possible and the HDL as high as possible, the best "risk ratio" numbers are the lowest (like a golf score).

What about triglycerides? What do they have to do with the price of hamburger?

Triglycerides are yet another member of the circulating fat molecule club, but one whose numbers vary dramatically depending upon the timing (and size) of the last meal, in addition to weight, diabetes, and genetics. A combination of high triglyceride levels and low HDL cholesterol appears to represent a specific, independent risk for coronary disease (usually with genetic underpinnings). Extremely high triglyceride levels are also a risk factor for pancreatitis, which can be a very serious illness.

So when I have a blood test for cholesterol, I need to find out more than just the total level, right?

Exactly. Your levels of total cholesterol, HDL, LDL, and triglycerides should be as important to you as your personal income. To be accurate, the blood should be drawn while you are fasting—that is, at least fourteen hours after the previous meal—because triglyceride levels (which affect measurements of the others) rise immediately after food.

So what if I find out that my numbers aren't so great? How can I change them?

In a nutshell, elevated LDL cholesterol and triglyceride levels usually respond to reducing fatty foods and increasing complex carbohydrates in the diet, a topic we have just discussed. This should be the first, last, and continuous order of business if the cholesterol levels are found to be unfavorable. Even if medication needs to be added to the mix at some point, maintaining optimal food choices is still the mainstay of treatment. Furthermore, the twenty-five grams of fiber per day takes on new significance, because these substances help reduce daily absorption of cholesterol.

Weight reduction is as important as the avoidance of fatty foods, assuming one is heavier than appropriate. Usually, in fact, the two go together, because the high-fat fuel is a lot more calorie-dense than the low-fat food. But it *is* possible to eat enough low fat food to keep the scales from dropping, in which case cholesterol may stay put, even in the face of seemingly heroic dietary efforts.

What about raising HDL? Wouldn't that be helpful?

Absolutely, but selectively raising it (without bringing LDL along for the ride) is a bit trickier. In fact, it cannot be done reliably even with the best food choices. Fortunately, HDL *does* tend to rise with regular exercise, which provides yet another good reason to begin an aerobics program.

What about using drugs to improve cholesterol?

This is a touchy subject for many people, because intuitively it seems that one ought to be able to improve the lipid landscape by making better food choices. And, in fact, changing what enters one's mouth can make a profound difference. But some people genetically have been dealt a hand which keeps cholesterol and/or triglycerides in the stratosphere, even with the most disciplined and appropriate diet. Others, even with the best coaching, simply cannot or will not make the necessary changes.

If lipid levels are high enough to represent a significant risk for coronary disease—especially if there are other risk factors on the table as well—starting medication may be an appropriate decision. (The same logic is commonly applied to the treatment of elevated blood pressure and is accepted much more widely, probably because fewer people believe that they can control blood pressure themselves.)

If I am to take medication to lower cholesterol or triglycerides, am I looking at a long-term proposition?

In general, yes. But sometimes the hassle and cost of taking pills serves as a motivater to make some necessary lifestyle changes, which in turn bring the numbers down far enough to stop the drugs.

Aren't there side-effects and risks to this sort of treatment?

Absolutely. No drug of any kind is totally risk-free. But, fortunately, the treatment for lipids usually isn't worse than the disease. Your doctor can give you a run-down of the options if medical treatment is necessary for you.

The fifth point on the checklist is closely related to the issues we've just discussed.

5. Deal with your blood pressure if it's elevated.

High blood pressure over prolonged periods of time is associated with an increased risk for some unsavory consequences: coronary artery disease, congestive heart failure, stroke, and kidney damage. Unfortunately, blood pressure is otherwise silent—no symptoms, no discomfort, no fatigue, just the disabling or deadly outcomes.

Wait a minute. I've talked to people who can tell when their blood pressure is high.

Frequently people will assume that a headache, heart pounding, or some other sensation of tension is caused by high blood pressure. Actually the opposite is true: pressure will go up in response to our being in pain, or tense, or uncomfortable (hence the familiar problem of "white coat hypertension," blood pressure elevated in the doctor's office but not other settings). Only at astronomical levels do symptoms develop directly from the blood pressure.

I thought the word hypertension referred primarily to one's mental condition.

The term refers only to levels of blood pressure, whether one is relaxed or needing to be scraped off the ceiling. Similarly, those with normal and low pressure are referred to as *normotensive* and *hypotensive* respectively.

But doesn't being anxious and tense cause high blood pressure?

It can certainly contribute, but genetics, weight, diet, exercise patterns, age, and certain medical conditions are also factors. Very often, unfortunately, hypertension is found to be *idiopathic*—a medical term that means "we dunno."

What levels should I be concerned about?

Blood pressure is measured in millimeters of mercury, the same units the weatherman uses to read the barometer. Each contraction of the heart produces a peak in pressure referred to as "systolic," and in between contractions the pressure falls to a low known as "diastolic." Ideally the systolic should stay below 140 and the diastolic below 90. The number is read as "(systolic) over (diastolic)" and written as (systolic)/(diastolic)—for example, 120/80.

Is one more important than the other?

At various times in the past, one or the other has been singled out as particularly important, but neither should be ignored. However, some allowances are made for elevation of the systolic pressure with advanced age.

What should I do if I get a reading above the recommended levels?

It depends on the level. If you are higher than 160 systolic or 105 diastolic, you should see your physician promptly for confirmation, further evaluation, and treatment. If the elevation is milder, it is helpful to get a few more readings on your own if possible, and then bring those to your doctor. Because blood pressure can vary considerably, decisions must be made based on trends rather than one or two readings. In fact, some people have what is called "labile" hypertension—their readings swing all over the map, depending on circumstances. Treatment decisions are definitely trickier in such cases.

What can I do about my blood pressure if it's elevated?

Again, this will hinge on the severity of the problem and other factors which have to be reviewed with your doctor. But some basic steps will help, at least to some degree:

1. Lose weight if you need to. (Notice how this keeps coming up....)

2. Begin an appropriate exercise program. (Notice how this keeps coming up as well....)

3. Curtail your intake of salt, whether dumped from the

shaker or laced in foods such as pickles, chips, many canned soups, and quite a few fast food entrees. The added sodium causes fluid to be increased and retained, and the added volume in the bloodstream increases pressure. (One of the tried and true blood pressure treatments, and the first line of therapy until a few years ago, is the diuretic or "water pill" which contracts the body's fluid volume.)

4. Take a look at your alcohol intake. Excessive alcohol, rather than having a physiologic calming effect, causes blood pressure to become erratic.

5. Take a look also at your current stress levels. If you feel as though your life is a continuous left turn against heavy traffic, a sprint across an eight-lane freeway where there are no safety zones, or a constant illustration of "out of the frying pan, into the fire," your autonomic nervous system may be on overdrive. Dealing with the issues of life is rarely a quick-fix proposition, and some serious discussions with a pastor, counselor, or even good friends may be in order.

At what point would I have to consider medication?

If your hypertension is mild (less than 160 systolic and/or 100 diastolic) some observation over time, while attempting some appropriate lifestyle changes, is adequate. But if this is unsuccessful after a few months, or if the pressure is cruising well beyond these levels, medication can protect you from prolonged exposure to hazardous pressures and their consequences.

But I've heard that once you start blood pressure medication, you can never get off. I wouldn't want to take pills the rest of my life.

Nor would anyone. Starting medication, however, is not always a sentence to lifetime use. The initial choices, adjustments, and ongoing refills will depend on a host of factors, including the progress of blood pressure over time. If an ongoing course of medical intervention appears necessary, there is such a wide variety of treatment options that you should be able to find a particular medication which works, can be taken only once or twice a day, and is essentially "invisible"—not causing any noticeable side effects. Twenty years ago it was likely that controlling blood pressure also meant feeling perpetually weary or stuporous, but that is not the case today.

6. Get the smoke out of your life.

To no one's great surprise, tobacco use has now been officially ranked as the number one underlying cause of death in the United States. Even though the actual leading killers may be heart disease and cancer, cigarettes (and to a lesser degree, other forms such as chewing tobacco) set these diseases in motion more often than any other factor. A major 1993 study from the Office of Disease Prevention at the U.S. Department of Health and Human Services, the first on fundamental causes of death, indicates that tobacco contributed to the deaths of 400,000 people in 1990.

**Not to wave a red flag in front of a bull, but how many
different kinds of problems does smoking
create or aggravate?**

The list of new diseases and misery literally grows every month: cancers of the lung, mouth, larynx, esophagus, uterine cervix, and bladder; chronic obstructive lung disease; heart attacks, and a higher risk of sudden death when these occur; peptic ulcer disease; tooth decay; osteoporosis; clogging of the arteries to the legs, resulting in pain on walking, or outright loss of toes, feet, or entire limbs; more frequent upper respiratory infections; infertility; multiple problems during pregnancy... not to mention bad breath, holes in clothes, risks of accidental fires, the smell of stale smoke throughout car and home, and harm to everyone in the vicinity who must breathe the smoke as well!

If tobacco use is such a big risk, why do people still smoke?

Smoking is a particularly intense form of drug addiction which happens to be legal, and it is supported by a $3 billion annual advertising budget from the tobacco industry. People start to smoke to look sophisticated, answer a dare, act out, or look tough. But once well established through repeated nicotine "hits" into the bloodstream and thousands of psychological connections to everyday activities (getting in the car, having coffee, answering the phone, etc.), the desire to smoke completely bypasses rational thinking and even overt discomfort. The choke-chain tenacity of this habit is well known to any physician who has tried to convince someone to quit in the face of a racking cough, shortness of breath, or even an outright lung cancer.

So how do people ever quit?

Some are able to make a deliberate decision one day, throw away the pack and never smoke again. Others must work through a weaning process, take classes, use nicotine replacements or other drugs, and even obtain counseling and tranquilizers. What helps in general are the following:
1. A written list of reasons. A desire not to be sick or dead before one's time; to preserve the one body we have been given for our time on earth; to live long enough to see grandchildren or complete a lifelong project; and so on.
2. Some emotion behind the decision. Sometimes this is provided by a good scare—a suspicious chest X-ray or a smok-

ing friend who contracts cancer. Or it may arise from the humiliating sense of being enslaved to some dried leaves wrapped in white paper. Or perhaps the realization that the tobacco industry continues to make huge profits in the face of the untold misery caused by its products.

3. A public declaration that one has quit. Most of us will work hard to avoid looking like a wimp after making our intentions known to others.

4. Completely eliminating all smoking products and paraphernalia from home, car, and work area.

5. Declaring home to be a smoke-free zone. This means that any smokers at home will have to indulge their habit outside or in the garage.

6. A stop-smoking class. These are available in most communities through local chapters of the American Lung Association.

7. A nicotine substitute, if withdrawal symptoms (irritability, restlessness) are difficult to manage.

Do these substitutes actually work?

They can make the quitting process smoother for some people. Nicorette®, the nicotine-laden gum, can help hold down the craving to a manageable level. The most popular modality at the moment is the nicotine patch, which releases this chemical slowly over several hours and maintains a steady blood level. These provide a buffer against withdrawal symptoms but without the pleasurable "hit" that occurs from a drag on a cigarette. (The patches occasionally irritate the skin, and all directions must be followed exactly.) To be successful, these products should be used every day for eight to twelve weeks, in order to allow enough time to break the connection between everyday activities and lighting up. A stop-smoking class taken during the same time period greatly increases the odds of long-term success.

What about the staple in the ear that's supposed to act like a prolonged acupuncture treatment?

Some smokers claim these have helped them quit, but we believe this represents self-fulfilling prophecy. Since this treatment isn't typically cheap, the smoker has basically made a multi-hundred dollar bet that the staple will kill the urge to light up. No one wants to see that much cash go up in smoke, and success (at least for a while) can result.

Overall, the best approaches to quitting do not involve magic potions or passive treatments but, like anything else in life that needs revision, require an honest look at the costs, dangers, and personal needs that are driving the habit.

What about the effects of other people's smoke on my health?

The EPA has officially listed "second-hand smoke" as a health hazard, primarily for respiratory disease, and you should make every effort to keep it out of your airspace. If your husband or other relatives smoke, they need to be banished to the yard if they feel they must light up. And under no circumstances should you have to breathe someone's cigarette exhaust at the workplace. Community and state laws are now increasingly stringent about this matter, and you are quite within your rights to bring this up with your employer if necessary.

7. Adjust your alcohol intake.

I assume you mean downward.

Naturally... assuming you drink alcohol, of course. Excessive alcohol consumption is a major risk to life and limb. The list of medical problems tied to alcohol is lengthy: aside from the well-known liver damage, it can contribute to diseases of the stomach, pancreas, heart, and nervous system. It plays a role in a variety of cancers, including mouth, throat, larynx, and liver. It can permanently damage the fetus if consumed by a pregnant woman.

How much would be considered excessive?

In terms of pure volume, anything more than one or two drinks per 24-hour period. A "drink" in this context is defined as a twelve-ounce beer, a four-ounce glass of wine, or a cocktail containing one ounce of distilled spirits. But the definition of "excess" has to include some other behaviors as well. Drinking is an issue if it has played a part in any disturbance within a family or with other people, loss of time from work, legal problem, or injury. It is a problem if, even on a rare occasion, a drink turns into a binge. It must be dealt with if it cannot be approached with a "take it or leave it" attitude. Anything resembling emotional attachment to alcohol is trouble.

Is there any benefit to alcohol use?

A number of studies have suggested that those who consume one or two drinks per day have fewer coronary events and fewer problems with gallstones than abstainers. But some newer research also suggests that this "moderate" use may increase the risk for cancer of the breast and colon.

There may be some medical rationale, therefore, for a modest intake (such as glass of wine with dinner) for someone with cardiac risk factors, such a strong family history of coronary artery disease or a high cholesterol level. But this may have to be weighed against one's risks for breast and colon cancer (see Chapter Seven for more details), as well as other personal and medical factors. In general, either abstention or infrequent use of modest amounts is the safest bet.

What if alcohol is, in fact, a problem?

The biggest hurdle is, without a doubt, acknowledging that there *is* in fact a problem with drinking. Once the denial has been breached, the two most important words are *get help*. Overcoming alcohol overuse is not for "Lone Rangers," and a combination of personal and group support is indispensable. Many churches now run Twleve Step programs or other structured activities which bring God explicitly into the recovery process.

8. Wear your seat belt.

Sounds like Mom's talking again. Is this a book on menopause or driver safety?

Actually you won't have to worry about hot flashes (or much else) if you're in a coma or six feet under. Several thousand deaths every year result from unbelted passengers making an unscheduled flight through the windshield of a car. And nearly as tragic are the myriad cases of permanent brain damage. Buckling up is a quick, easy action which can prevent an incredible amount of distress for yourself and those you love.

9. Keep your sex life a "closed system."

The biblical mandate for sex is for one man and one woman to maintain a publicly committed, mutually exclusive marital relationship—a closed system into which sexually transmitted organisms have no access. This also happens to be the only way to have truly "safe" sex. And, if universally followed, it would end an unprecedented epidemic of several disabling and lethal diseases. The same study which attributed 400,000 deaths to tobacco use in 1990 also linked about 30,000 to sexual behavior that same year.

But why bring this up in a book about menopause?

While it is common to think of sexually transmitted diseases (STDs) as a particular concern of the young, the bacteria and viruses that cause syphilis, gonorrhea, pelvic inflammatory disease, hepatitis B, cancer of the cervix, and AIDS don't know or care how old you are. In fact, as of June, 1993, more than 5,500 women in the U.S. with AIDS are forty-five or older (about 13 percent of the total female population with this disease). As we will explore in depth later, sexuality does not retire with the last menstrual period—nor does the importance of safeguarding and expressing this gift within the proper context.

What's this about cancer of the cervix?

Glad you noticed. The human papilloma virus (HPV), which is sexually transmitted, is clearly implicated in the development of the changes that lead to cervical cancer—which, by the way, kills far more women every year than AIDS. This is why early sexual experience and multiple sexual partners are well-known risk factors for this tumor.

What about hepatitis B? I thought that was spread through IV drug use and contaminated blood transfusions.

And through sexual intercourse. In fact, researchers recognized early on in the AIDS epidemic that the populations that acquired this disease were similar to those with hepatitis B, leading to the hypothesis—and eventual identification—of a virus (now well known as HIV, or human immunodeficiency virus) as the underlying cause. The hepatitis B virus, by the way, infects 300,000 Americans every year, and 1.2 million are chronic carriers.

My friend's husband passed away a few years ago, and now she plans to remarry. How can she be sure her husband-to-be won't infect her with some disease, even though he feels well?

The question you raise, unfortunately, isn't merely academic (or paranoid). Most STDs are transmitted by people who have no idea they have been infected, perhaps years in the past. Hopefully, with a marriage on the horizon, your friend has gleaned by now some idea about her future spouse's past history and (even more importantly) his honesty. If he has had one or more sexual partners before her, and they were not "closed system" marriages, she might need to broach the delicate question of screening for a silent infection. (Obviously, the same could be said on his behalf regarding her.)

The most important STDs that can be identified through blood screening are syphilis (required in most states for the marriage license), HIV and hepatitis B (both of which *should* be required for the license). Other STDs are suspected more by history: recurrent, self-healing groups of blisters on the penis (herpes simplex); so-called "venereal warts" (HPV); a discharge from the penis at some time in the past (gonorrhea or chlamydia). A history of any of these events would best be discussed (individually or together) with a physician, since their present and future implications can vary greatly.

Wouldn't condoms protect me if my partner had one of these infections?

While condoms certainly reduce the risk of STD transmission, they are so far from foolproof that it is astonishing to see how much adulation they have received during the past few years. For many years condoms were considered the bottom of the barrel in contraceptive technology. Condom failure rates for preventing pregnancy are still widely accepted as being—at best—around 10 percent. That means one in ten women who are fertile and having intercourse regularly will become pregnant within a year if condoms are the only form of birth control they use. But an egg and sperm can only unite one or two days out of every month, while STDs can be transmitted any day of the year.

Some agencies are now claiming that condoms are 98 to 99 percent effective in preventing the spread of HIV, a number that is not supported by the bulk of medical literature on the subject, and certainly not applicable to pregnancy and sexually-transmitted diseases. However, condoms *can* be 100 percent effective when used correctly and consistently... as a bookmark.

* * *

You've spent an awful lot of time on these health issues which aren't specifically applicable to women in mid-life. What's the point?

These basic maintenance issues make a huge impact on the well-being of women of all ages, but especially in the years approaching and following menopause. All of the specific changes and issues related to the conclusion of the reproductive years play out against the background of this "state of the union." Furthermore, and more importantly, these are health concerns over which we all have a great deal of control. You cannot expect doctors, the EPA, any health care plan (comprehensive or otherwise), food supplements, or the good fairy to be responsible for your health or "make you well." If more than half of all deaths (and by implication a similar proportion of non-lethal health problems) are linked to the everyday decisions we have discussed, they are well worth reviewing, pondering, and—most of all—doing.

Chapter Four
꩜

How Do I Get Ready?
Part II: Relational, Intellectual, Emotional, and Spiritual Preparations

I have a question before we get started. Why is this chapter included in a book about menopause?

We believe that God purposefully created us in such a way that everything is interconnected. Physical problems affect our emotions. Emotional issues play a huge role in our physical health. And spiritual issues affect everything. If we only discussed medical issues, we'd be ignoring the rest of the puzzle.

OK, that makes sense to me. So where do we start?

Let's start with relationships. The middle years are usually a time of great upheaval in a woman's primary relationships. The dynamics between a woman and her aging parents, her newly grown children, and even her own husband change through a series of unavoidable adjustments.

RELATIONSHIPS WITH AGING PARENTS.

I'm just beginning to feel as though my responsibilities for my kids are ending, but now I see my parents needing more of my input and my time. Am I unusual in being unsettled by this development?

Not at all. When we began our own adult life, our parents served as dispensers of helpful advice (some of which was even *wanted*), bankers for emergency financing, havens of uncomplaining childcare, and providers of countless free meals. (National surveys have concluded that *no one* makes turkey stuffing like Teri's mom, or stroganoff like Paul's....)

Then, just as we hit the heavy responsibilities (and soul-searching) of the middle years, the base of security our parents have always represented begins to erode. At a time when we need their reassuring hugs and stabilizing effect, our parents' health starts to fail, and they no longer have the physical or emotional stamina of their younger years. The illness of one spouse becomes (rightfully) the full-time preoccupation of the other. And the death of a spouse can leave the surviving partner in a state of loneliness and emotional need, changing the directional flow of loving care from child to parent.

While we were in the process of writing this book, Teri's dad died of a sudden cerebral hemorrhage. Four years ago, he had been very active and healthy until two successive bouts with lung cancer left him in a weakened condition. It became strange and painful to watch this man, who had always been so physically fit, give up even his beloved golf game because its mild exertion left him winded. Since he has gone to be with the Lord he loved so much, Teri now feels her relationship with her mom changing to one of a more protective nature.

There is no practical way to prepare for this process. There are no warm-up exercises, no dry runs, and certainly no magic formula to predict the future. And, alas, there is no way that we, in a few pages, can cover the length and breadth of the relationships between parents and children. But a few basic attitudes cultivated over a period of years may make these transitions smoother.

First, if you have a good relationship with your parents, don't take it for granted. Just as we tend to think that our kids will never leave the land of dirty diapers and messy rooms—and then suddenly we find them heading out the door—so we are prone to expect our parents to live forever. Realize that their remaining years are numbered, and make time to be with them. This can be particularly challenging during the years when our agendas are the most crowded, when the demands on our own time are the most intense.

During the fall of 1993, Teri set aside several days out of her hectic schedule and flew home for a time of long conversations over morning coffee, bargain hunting at local factory outlets, several hotly contested games of Scrabble, and even an overnight "campout" in a newly acquired motor home. It was her best visit ever with her dad—and also her last. When he suddenly lost consciousness two months later, and it became clear he would never awaken, she was comforted with those recent, pleasant memories. His passing, and the subsequent memorial services, were times to appreciate and bond with other family members, rather than deal with floods of regrets.

That's all fine when you've had such a good relationship. But what if I'm not exactly warm and fuzzy with my parents at this point in my life? Why should I spend a lot of time and energy (and emotion) trying to get close to them now?

No law says you have to orchestrate a major reconciliation, assuming one is needed. But like it or not, parent-child relationships are extremely powerful forces in our lives, even long after we leave home. Having one or both depart this earth while there is enmity or a chilly gap remaining in your relationship can leave a major emotional wake. And, after a period of hostility or silence, reaching a point of mutual respect and even love can have a powerfully energizing effect on all concerned.

One of Paul's most difficult cases involved an extremely demented and debilitated elderly woman who was brought by her daughter to the emergency room on a chilly December 26 many years ago. The woman could respond to voices and touch only with moans and an oddly sweet smile. Her limbs were permanently flexed from lack of movement, and over each hip a huge pressure sore had eroded through skin into what little fat remained below it. Barely able to swallow, she was acutely ill, dehydrated, and probably septic (with bacteria circulating through the bloodstream). This was not exactly the most pleasant post-Christmas package, and her daughter's agenda made the situation even more difficult. Usually in such cases, loved ones will ask that the medical caregivers not go overboard, but do what they can to "make Mom comfortable" while nature takes its course. But here the mandate was quite different: "Do whatever is necessary to get Mom well."

Not knowing this family at all, and full of youthful compliance and fervor, Paul plunged ahead, bringing all his medical expertise to bear on this very frail patient. In spite of repeated hospitalizations and a variety of treatments, the woman's health continued to fail. The daughter was angry and distraught that "more wasn't being done," while colleagues of Paul's were quietly asking him why he was "flogging this poor patient," going overboard with aggressive treatments in a futile situation.

Finally, all the doctors involved in the case, along with a social worker, met with the daughter. They carefully reviewed the patient's numerous medical problems, having set the stage first with an eloquent description of the advanced consequences of aging and dementia that could never be reversed. Finally the daughter, a woman in her mid-fifties, broke down and wept. Her mother, she explained, had for decades been relentlessly cold and critical. But as her intellectual prowess declined, she had softened; and when her mental faculties failed, she had become openly affectionate. This poignant and ironic situation had tapped into all of her daughter's still unmet need for parental affection—hence the determination to keep Mom alive at all cost.

You may have some major unresolved issues—including anger and bitterness over negligence, innocent mistakes, or outright wrongs your parents have committed against you—which need to be dealt with before you can heal a wounded relationship. We suggest discussing these issues with someone you can trust—a pastor, counselor, or mature friend. If the pains from your childhood are intense and pervasive, you would be wise to seek some outside counsel before attempting reconciliation. Christian counseling can be extremely helpful in resolving the hurts of the past and discovering God's healing love.

It is possible to obey God's command to honor one's parents even while bringing up some painful issues. If you are ready to discuss these issues with your parents, one approach to consider is putting your thoughts and feelings in writing. This gives you a chance to express yourself without becoming tongue-tied or out of control. You can review it, pray over it, and share it with someone you trust before sending it. Ideally, your written statement can be geared as an invitation to dialogue, whether on paper or in person, rather than serving as a vengeful artillery blast. Acknowledging your own shortcomings in the relationship can bring down some defenses as well. But if conversations are opened, barriers breached, sins confessed and forgiven, and affection rekindled, few events in your life will be as great a balm to the soul.

As you contemplate the failings in the relationship with your parents, remember one important point: the fact that your parents didn't effectively communicate their love for you does not mean they didn't love you. Most likely, they were passing on the patterns that they were given. It is quite possible that your parents have loved you fiercely, but they also have come from a family or era in which affection was not freely given or received.

Unfortunately, not every attempt at reaching out will be successful. While you can make an honest effort, you cannot engineer the results. The response you receive may be cool, hostile, or absent. But the apostle Paul instructed us that "if it is possible, *as far as it depends on you*, live at peace with everyone"—including, we can be sure, our own parents (Rom. 12:18, emphasis added). If you have gone as far as you can, you will avoid dealing with the same regrets that plague those who have let the sun set on their anger for years.

RELATIONSHIPS WITH GROWING AND GROWN-UP CHILDREN.

I've been hearing from a few friends about the "empty nest" syndrome. Is this a pop psychology concoction or a real problem I should be preparing for?

With rare exception, letting go of grown children is an emotional event, one for which many parents—especially moms—have not prepared. In order to maintain balance and sanity, it is critical that we see parenthood as a process of gradually giving children greater independence (and at times having them wrench some of it away from us), as they pass from the first squirming days of total need to that inevitable day when our home is no longer their base of operations. In a best case scenario, we experience a smooth transition from carrying total responsibility for a child to enjoying a relaxed friendship with an independent adult. In two worst case scenarios, the parenting job never comes to a close, or a parent feels a devastating loss of purpose and worth when the last child goes out the door.

When our own two children were strewing toys and spilling milk, we used to dream of the day that our house would be all ours once again. We were more than happy to let them spend a weekend with Gramma and Grampa occasionally. (Our children were blessed with grandparents who savored that role and who cherished them.) But when our son Chad charged into his senior year of high school and began planning his first year away at college, we found ourselves fighting an unnamed but recurring uneasiness.

Of course, we were excited about this prospect. But suddenly we also had a powerful reminder of our limited time remaining with him, and a sense of loss as his circle of friends and interests continued to expand. And there seemed to be so *much* we had yet to instill in him. (He still didn't know how to iron a shirt properly, for Pete's sake!) But, ready or not, the time was fast approaching, and he would soon be making all his own decisions. His transition has given us a heightened awareness that the remaining two years with daughter Carrie at home are to be savored, for they will be fleeting.

So, for better or worse, no matter how many kids we bring into the world, the job of parenting children will eventually be OVER. Our responsibilities—looking out for their needs, teaching, setting limits, discipline, and even the nighttime rituals—sooner or later come to an end. Children are, after all, only loaned to us by their Creator for a season. And the close of that season can leave a huge, yawning hole in the life of the woman who has never developed her own interests and talents while sacrificially devoting every extra moment to home and family. This can be even more of an issue for the woman who had to work outside the home and then felt too guilty to take away any *more* time from the family by attending classes, developing a hobby, or joining a women's support group or Bible study.

What happens to the woman whose children no longer need her after eighteen years of worrying, loving, nagging, disciplining, cleaning, and cooking? There is a natural tendency to feel unappreciated and abandoned... which is why we badger women to begin developing a few of their own interests after the children are into their school years. A woman can establish her own interests and identity without moving the family from its rightful place as the number one priority. Then, when the middle years abruptly arrive, a woman has a foundation of other interests to which she can now devote more time.

But if you are already at this "empty nest" stage and are starting at ground zero, don't despair! Just understand that some of the depression you may be currently experiencing might be grief for the big chunk of your identity which has been removed. As we will discuss in the next section, this is a perfect time to redefine your worth in terms of whose *child* you are (God's) rather than whose mom you are. This change in orientation is more than just an abstraction. The woman who can't emotionally release her grown children is the woman who becomes embroiled in details with which she has no business being concerned. The woman with no life of her own can become the legendary mother-in-law who becomes the butt of nasty jokes because she is obsessed with continuing to influence her children's lives long after they are grown.

What about the other end of the spectrum? In these days of job scarcity and high costs of living, I've also been hearing about parents who can't seem to get their kids out on their own.

Some grown children aren't eager to leave comfortable living quarters. Because of rising costs of education, many high school graduates are forced to live at home while attending the local junior college. Because of astronomical housing prices, some young married couples spend their first several months in Mom and Dad's guest room. Worse yet is the twenty-something "adult" who can't seem to figure out what to do, and thus vegetates at home for what seems an eternity while the bewildered parents wonder what went wrong.

If a grown child is to remain at home, two very important issues need to be considered. First, this arrangement must be mutually agreeable! It's one thing to let the kids know that the porch light will always be on; but permission needs to be granted for the door to remain unlocked.

Second, and more important, the relationship between parent and adult child must be redefined. Because this is a time in which your son or daughter should be individuating *away* from you, you need to facilitate this process by subtly (and sometimes not so subtly) demanding that he or she function as an adult. This includes treating parents and their hard-earned property with respect, being responsible for their own expenses (including kicking in a little cash toward the food bill and rent), doing their own laundry and dishes, etc. In other words, grown children must live in the house with the status of an adult boarder, albeit a beloved one. A mom who continues to allow her grown child to act as if he or she were still in high school is granting no great favors; in fact, she is thwarting emotional maturity and guaranteeing perpetual frustration for all.

The flip side of this, Mom, is that you can no longer treat your son or daughter as if you're still in charge of making all the decisions! You don't set study hours, tell your daughter what to wear, or pass judgment on whom your son should date. You do have the right, however, to establish and enforce codes of conduct under your own roof. One of our favorite kitchen magnets reads as follows:

HOUSE RULES

1. We own the house.
2. We make the rules.

If your children are making some bad decisions about smoking, drinking, sex, or disorderly conduct, you can't force them to conform to your standards of right and wrong. But you have every right to insist that, if they continue indulging in unacceptable behaviors, they do it elsewhere. And if clearly understood house rules are being broken repeatedly, it's important to give notice to your "boarder" and then send them on the way, just as you would do with anyone else sharing your space. We have both counseled bewildered parents who are struggling with disruptive, disrespectful, or even abusive adult offspring. But when the offenses are taking place on the parent's home turf, there can be only one course of action: a decisive boot out the door, no matter how "unloving" it might seem, and no matter what (legal) measures are necessary. Keep in mind that it is not a manifestation of love to facilitate someone's self-destructive or anti-social behavior.

On the other hand, if house rules are respected, and there is a conscious shift from a parenting mode to a "benevolent landlady" mode, then this potentially difficult situation can be quite pleasant and mutually beneficial. You might even become friends with your child—something that doesn't normally happen until a little physical distance separates you!

RELATING TO YOUR HUSBAND

I'm not so concerned about falling apart once the kids leave. But I feel like I don't have nearly as much in common with my husband as I did twenty years ago. Frankly,

I'm a little nervous about the prospects of being "just a couple" again. Am I overreacting?

It depends on the amount of repair work your marriage needs. Unfortunately, the middle years are a prime time for divorce in this country. A couple can mask marital difficulties quite successfully during the busy childrearing years. In fact, whenever a parent brings a child in for counseling, one of the first things a family therapist will seek to discover are the problems between Mom and Dad which are being carefully ignored while "all hands are on deck" tending to the child who is acting out. But when the children are no longer in the picture on a daily basis, a couple cannot avoid looking at the unresolved issues which lie between them.

One of the worst situations for a middle-aged woman to face is a husband who is completely apathetic toward her—because apathy, not hate, is the opposite of love. Unfortunately, it is impossible to build a relationship when only one person is willing to participate. If you find yourself in this sad situation, we do not encourage you to leave the marriage because divorce has devastating repercussions at any stage. Rather, we suggest that you build up your female friendships to meet your need for companionship and support, do what you can to breathe new life into the relationship, and begin working on your personal issues.

The scenario with a better prognosis is one where strong feelings are still being experienced, even if they are negative. If you are verbally fighting with your husband, and he's upset enough to seek marriage counseling with you, there is plenty of hope that stress-provoking issues can be resolved. (A word of warning—when a verbal argument progresses to property damage or physical abuse of *any* kind, (defined as the use of any kind of violence or physical coercion), it is an *immediate* signal for a time of separation of at least three to six months.

During this time, participating in professional marital counseling must be one of the conditions for moving back together.)

Much of the work in this type of situation will lie in changing the communication patterns. Many couples spend a lifetime sharpening their verbal rapier blades and defending their personal strongholds from volleys of hurtful words. The nicest gift anyone can give to a newlywed couple is a "couples' communication class," where a husband and wife learn how to transmit information and share feelings in a manner that is both effective and mutually respectful. But it is *never* too late to learn how to communicate if you have a willing partner. A major act of optimistic courage would be to locate such a class in your community and give it to your husband as a Christmas, birthday, Valentine's Day, Groundhog Day, or any day gift. If no such class can be found, grab some of your favorite married couples and start your own by using either *Talking Together* (by Sherod Miller, Elam W. Nunnally, and Daniel B. Wackman) or *Messages* (by Matthew McKay, Martha Davis, and Patrick Fanning).

I'm not worried about a trench war at home as much as a deadly silence. What can I do to prevent this from happening?

For too many couples, the daily details of raising kids can obliterate the companionship and camaraderie that got the relationship (and the kids) going in the first place. Equally numbing are separate career tracks which evolve into distant orbits around other people and projects. Without some deliberate maintenance, such a marriage turns into a stale cohabitation, with the added risk that either party might slide into an affair.

Just as your body cannot be maintained in optimal condition without some proactive lifestyle decisions, neither can your marriage flourish if it is not given some deliberate attention and nurturing. At the risk of sounding like a well-worn cookbook, we feel it is important to toss out some "basic maintenance" concepts for your marriage as well.

1. Remember what got you started, and celebrate it. You don't need an anniversary to sit down with those old photo albums or even pay a visit to the places where the sparks first were lit. We never tire of reminiscing about the intense romance of our first months together, both before and after the wedding ceremony. Our kids moan and groan when we get started, but that's tough. And they actually confess to a sense of security when they hear us savoring some steamy remembrance of our early days.

2. Talk between yourselves.

That's easy for you to say. My husband is the proverbial "man of few words," especially at the end of the day. How do I get him to open up to me instead of the evening paper?

Take him out to dinner, or to breakfast if he's truly exhausted after the work day, or wait until the weekend. And then start asking questions and showing interest. Do you have any idea what his work is all about, what issues he's dealing with every day, what he's thinking about? This shouldn't be an inquisition, but a flattering display of interest in *him,* not just the paycheck he brings home. Remember: feeling important and interesting is a powerful force of attraction. You should be the one who corners the market in this area. The Book of Proverbs, in a rich cautionary tale, describes how a disastrous adultery begins with flattery, not sexual lust (Prv 7:21).

3. Get away for a night or two.

Again, easy for you to say. Our schedules are socked in for weeks....

All the more reason to make this effort at least twice a year. If you have to, look far enough ahead in both of your calendars to a blank spot, put a big X across it, and tell him he's yours for those one or two nights. You plan it the first time, and make it worth his while. Chances are he'll want to put together the next one.

What if we can't afford a weekend of bon-bons and caviar at the Ritz?

Who says we're talking about a financial hemorrhage? The point is to be away from the endless demands and brush fires that distract you from one another. The setting needs to be pleasant but not extravagant, and (if possible) distant enough from home to allow the tugs of daily responsibilities to fade away for a while.

Bed and breakfast spots can be particularly relaxing, and most bookstores and libraries contain guidebooks describing inns in your area. Don't forget that off-season rates can be amazingly affordable. Many Christian conference centers rent rooms or cabins to couples, and may throw in meals as well, for even lower rates. For those who are truly limited in budget, find another couple in the same boat and switch houses for a weekend, just to get a change of scenery!

The object is to have time to linger over a meal, take walks, wander through some shops if any are in the neighborhood, read together for pure enjoyment, take an afternoon nap without feeling guilty, rub each other's feet, backs, and other body parts, and most of all get re-acquainted.

4. Get into a couples' group. Many churches have a network of small groups that meet during the week. In fact, much of the real ministry takes place in these settings, which can allow so much more interaction than the standard "Hihowzitgoing, Godblessyou" on Sunday morning. Ideally, these are not merely Bible studies in which a teacher stands in a living room and addresses the assembled few for an hour or more. In the best situations, Scripture is blended with discussion, openness, needs and issues, encouragement, exhortation, problem solving, prayer and (when necessary) an occasional loving confrontation—assuming that those involved trust each other enough. If biblical teaching is to interact with the trench wars of everyday life, this is the preparation area.

We have a hard enough time opening up to one another when we're on our own... I don't think we're ready for this group stuff.

Hey, this isn't taking off your clothes and jumping into a hot tub with eight other people. The process of getting comfortable and involved in a group doesn't happen in one evening. You might consider joining with another couple or two that you already know. But if that isn't possible, and the get-together reminds you of a group blind date, there's nothing wrong with taking a relaxed approach for a while, chiming in when either one of you feels ready. You can even make a polite departure if the chemistry doesn't work after an honest effort. But when a group hits its stride, offering trust, support, personal repair work, and relaxed fun, the weekly get-together can become an oasis and a support for your marriage.

5. Get into a common project that involves just the two of you. Whether a hobby, some form of recreation, or a full-blown ministry project, working side-by-side in any endeavor has a way of stimulating conversation and building new bonds. One of our favorite role models for this principle is a middle-aged couple in Southern California who manage a home for single pregnant women. They are not particularly wealthy or glamorous, and the problems they must solve together—from fixing appliances to trouble-shooting their way through their clients' various crises—are enormous. But their sense of shared purpose and cooperation is readily apparent to everyone around them.

* * *

You've spent a lot of time dealing with relationships involving a spouse and kids. What if there is no husband or kids as the menopause approaches and passes?

Many women are on their own as they press on through their mid-life years and beyond. Whether through divorce, untimely death of a husband, never having connected with the right person, or singleness by choice, the absence of a partner may be more acutely felt at this time than ten or twenty years ago. And if childless, the end of the reproductive years may prove a heavy milestone indeed. Menopause is also a difficult time for those women who have exerted much effort and emotion in unsuccessful attempts to become pregnant. (Some adventurous infertility researchers, it should be noted, are attempting to achieve pregnancy in women who are actually postmenopausal, using hormonal support and donor eggs. Such efforts are controversial, to say the least, moving deeply into some uncharted and choppy ethical waters.)

The Bible offers good news to the single adult, particularly in two key passages from the apostle Paul. (Paul admittedly was not a perimenopausal woman, but he nevertheless expressed ideas profoundly comforting and applicable to these situations). Writing from the most unsavory circumstances of a Philippian jail, he had the astonishing perspective to pen these familiar words:

I have learned to be content whatever the circumstances. I know what it is to be in need, and I know what it is to have plenty. I have learned the secret of being content in any and every situation, whether well fed or hungry, whether living in plenty or in want. I can do everything through him who gives me strength. Phil 4:11-13

We could easily extrapolate his list of circumstances for which contentment should be the primary state of mind: "...whether in a house full of kids or all by myself, whether at the peak of a career or with few skills, whether financially secure or living hand to mouth."

The other passage deals with the unmarried person's freedom to serve God:

I would like you to be free from concern. An unmarried man is concerned about the Lord's affairs—how he can please the Lord. But a married man is concerned about the affairs of this world—how he can please his wife—and his interests are divided. An unmarried woman or virgin is concerned about the Lord's affairs: Her aim is to be devoted to the Lord in both body and spirit. But a married woman is concerned about the affairs of this world—how she can please her husband. I am saying this for your own good, not to restrict you, but that you may live in a right way in undivided devotion to the Lord. 1 Cor 7:32-35

These are not sighs of resignation or sour grapes. Paul is simply stating a fact: when married, it is necessary to pay attention to that relationship. When not, it is possible to get involved in projects that might hinder a married couple, let alone one with children. Neither the married or the unmarried state is "better" or "worse" in God's economy: what matters in either condition is experiencing God's contentment, and from that powerful base, doing the most to advance his purposes.

Those who are in the best position to launch out for the great adventure of serving God in exotic situations are the unmarried or the married without kids (or with children who are launched into adulthood). If you aren't married or don't have the responsibilities of childrearing, your life can encompass some incredible experiences. Your most important job is getting so close to God that you see all circumstances—whether pleasing or challenging from the earthly vantage point—as part of a grand expedition that he has set before you.

INTELLECTUAL PREPARATIONS

Yeah, that's me—the intellectual. Who's got time for navel-contemplating when the daily to-do list never ends?

Whether you've been at home raising children for the past twenty years or working outside the home to help stretch the family budget, it's a fairly safe bet that you haven't spent the majority of your time doing the most stimulating tasks in the world. If you're one of the fortunate few who work in an environment that *does* cultivate your intellectual development, skip to the next section. The rest of you know precisely who you are, so turn off those "Mary Tyler Moore" reruns and tune in.

Here's the number one piece of advice for preparing yourself mentally for menopause: GO BACK TO SCHOOL! Now listen carefully, because we're not suggesting that everyone needs to have the goal of earning a degree. We're talking about taking just *one class at a time* in a few subjects which fascinate you. A world history survey, American history, art history or appreciation, music history or appreciation—anything of a "survey" nature is an excellent start. Some will enjoy tackling Psychology 101 in order to learn (or become totally confused about) why we "tick" the way we do.

You may not agree with the some of the viewpoints you hear, but that's OK. In fact, you may be the only person in the class with enough perspective and street-smarts to challenge the professor's biases. You may or may not decide to progress on toward a degree, but that's not the point. The idea is to put yourself in a situation where your brain is getting some exercise. Let's face it: it's all too easy to check out of the flow of stimulating ideas in order to raise our kids, and now is the best time to jump back into the stream.

I would love to go back and earn the degree I was never able to finish. But I just can't go back full-time. It'll take me ten years to finish my program! What's the use?

Barring unforeseen events, those ten years are going to pass whether you're working on your degree or not, correct? And you're going to be ten years older either with or without that degree, correct? Are you catching our drift? *So what* if it takes you years and years to finish—*the joy is in the process of growing!* One of Teri's role models is a woman who returned to school in her fifties, after her family was raised and gone. Now in her mid-seventies, she is a very successful psychologist in our community and a testimony to what can be accomplished in one's "later years."

But I feel so silly signing up for classes at my age— what will everyone think?

Wow, welcome to the 90s! Older students are flocking back to colleges and universities in droves these days, and professors usually *love* getting these students in their classes.

Why is that?

Because, while the 18-year-olds are thinking about what to wear to next weekend's party or how to get a "C" with the least amount of work, the older returning students are experiencing euphoria from the sheer joy of learning again. You will be a welcome addition to any class.

But I wouldn't have a clue how to begin.

Before she took a hiatus from school, Teri courageously negotiated her way around the huge UCLA campus, pregnant and with a toddler in tow. But when she decided to return to a small town campus and finish her undergrad work ten years later, those old confidence levels had plummeted. She felt as though her brain had dried up during the nursing period (as manifested by her continuing fascination with Big Bird, Bert, and Ernie long after the children were no longer interested in Sesame Street).

As she approached the registrar's office, she almost turned around and went back home. Fortunately, there are now so many returning women students that many campuses actually cater to them! This was the case in our town, and it made the difference in her staying and eventually completing her degree. So *ask* if your local college has someone in admissions who specializes in helping women like yourself integrate back into the system. It is very likely that someone on staff has this specific assignment. (One note of caution: if they steer you toward the campus Women's Center, be careful. This may prove to be a hotbed of radical feminist ideology rather than an oasis for *all* of the female students.)

But what about those who don't have a college anywhere nearby and are not sure they'd have the time to do a whole course even if they did?

A couple of suggestions include looking into correspondence courses from a more distant college or university. Working alone takes discipline, of course, so you might want to consider doing it with a friend. Or how about devising a reading program for yourself by asking the local high school for a "top 100" list of books students should read prior to graduation, and then go down the list systematically? Better yet, find one or more other women in need of some intellectual expansion and form a book club that meets weekly to discuss a book.

And don't limit your mental exercise to book work. Journaling your thoughts, your earliest memories, and your observations about the details or the grand sweep of life can be not only stimulating but possibly a joy or a help to someone else. Paul has been writing, at a very leisurely pace, some memoirs of his childhood and giving them to his mom in installments. (Paul's mom has retaliated with a detailed and funny account of his birth.) The same could be done for a good friend or one of your kids. Your material might even find its way into print some day. After all, Erma Bombeck and Dave Barry have entertained millions of people by describing everyday events with a keen and wry edge.

Your flow of ideas to paper, of course, doesn't have to be limited to chronicling what's going on in your head or your home. Short stories, novels, children's books, and poetry may all be rattling around in your imagination, waiting to be written. (Christian Writers Conferences are a wonderful place to learn and to meet other interesting people.) Don't forget that the entire multi-million dollar "Barney" phenomenon began because two moms decided there wasn't enough video material which their toddlers could enjoy.

EMOTIONAL/SPIRITUAL PREPARATIONS

Why are you linking these areas together?

We have combined these two components of the total picture because it is so difficult to influence one without affecting the other. In his letter to the Galatians, the apostle Paul contrasted the consequences of submission to the Spirit of God with those arising from our rebellious nature. The first (better known as "fruit of the Spirit,") primarily includes positive emotions and their by-products: love, joy, peace, patience, kindness, goodness, faithfulness, gentleness, and self-control. The others ("acts of the sinful nature," as he calls them) include not only destructive behaviors, but also a number of negative emotional states: hatred, jealousy, fits of rage, envy, and so on (Gal 5:19-23). And in between these two extremes are a multitude of emotional states and shadings which interact closely with our spiritual condition.

To avoid any misunderstanding, we should note that we do not endorse either of two extreme notions. First, some authors imply that every unpleasant emotion is a spiritual issue. This may produce shallow or oversimplified responses to problems such as depression: "You just need to pray more," or "Just memorize this passage of Scripture," for example. Such remedies obviously won't hurt, and may be important ingredients to recovery, but they may also ignore some crucial realities of human psychology and biochemistry, which we will explore in the next chapter.

The second extreme idea is that emotionalism equates to godliness. This leads to the dangerous presumption that frothing ecstasy or torrents of tears are the only manifestations of spiritual maturity. Intense emotions certainly will occur at times during an ongoing relationship with God, as they will in any important relationship. But to count on them, demand them, or generate them artificially displays at best a

misunderstanding of God and at worst an emotional incontinence that will turn off everyone in the vicinity.

Nevertheless, to restate our opening premise, there is a
direct and continuous interplay between one's emotional and
spiritual status. The condition of one's relationship with God
will influence the emotional weather for days, weeks, or a lifetime; and ongoing emotional difficulties can seriously interfere with that relationship as well.

**What you're talking about is not unique to any one
period of life. Is there any issue that particularly affects
women around menopause?**

The mid-life years for most people are a period of personal
re-evaluation, including some form of spiritual assessment.
The approach and completion of a woman's final reproductive cycle is a major milestone, which can (and should) provoke a review of life's progress and her spiritual "state of the
union." She may begin to ponder the reality that her physical
body has a meter running, to feel some concern over what
happens when time is up, and to wonder if her life has really
counted for anything. In doing so she will find herself somewhere on a very wide spectrum.

**Somewhere between a serial killer and
Mother Teresa, right?**

Actually, the spectrum does encompass good and evil, but
here we're thinking about an even more fundamental issue:
the status of one's basic relationship with God. From this
angle, the possibilities range from outright hostility on one
end to deep intimacy and fervent involvement on the other,
with gradations such as discomfort, indifference, sporadic
communication, or positive (if less than perfect) commitment
in between.

If someone has been completely disinterested in God up until now, isn't it a little late to start from scratch?

Not at all. Women who for years have shied away from discussions of "religion" may, at mid-life, find themselves on a serious quest for meaning. They may for the first time ask the most basic questions about God. Teri's experience in counseling demonstrates that even women who have studiously avoided church or synagogue have deep spiritual facets which they are eager to discuss under the right circumstances. In fact, this type of woman is usually refreshingly candid about spiritual issues because she hasn't been inoculated by years of tuning out during Sunday morning sermons!

If you are exploring these questions for the first time with your adult mind—a particularly important process if you rejected any childhood indoctrination of bygone years—we would encourage you to take a hard look at the teachings and claims of Jesus in the four Gospels. (And please, get a translation of the Bible, such as the New International Version, that is both accurate and written in contemporary English.)

Then consider the dilemma that C.S. Lewis described half a century ago: the teachings of Jesus are insightful, powerful, not to mention downright shrewd, but his claims about himself if false are those of a megalomaniac or a liar. Hopefully you will join the millions over the centuries who have come to the conclusion that he was not merely a popular (and then unpopular) rabbi, a brilliant teacher, or some blissed-out Mediterranean guru, but the literal entrance of God into the human race.

But beyond recognizing who Christ was (and is) comes a crucial step. We also must understand that he has solved the ultimate problem of every human being—that of estrangement from God because of personal rebellion (what the Scriptures call sin)—by dying, with horrendous suffering, in our place. Jesus, the one whose life was perfect and without fault, took the penalty that was due us. But in order to be free and clear we must individually acknowledge that our attitudes and conduct have indeed fallen well short of God's standards, articulated not just in the Ten Commandments but in Jesus' elaboration of them—which apply to all of us.

Furthermore, we need to understand that any efforts to earn God's favor through our own good works, rituals, or mental gyrations are totally futile, like an attempt to broad jump the Grand Canyon. And finally, we need to repent of our self-centered, self-justifying, self-serving ways and accept both God's forgiveness and ownership of our lives. That event occurs at a point in time, but its consequences are eternal. And when such an event truly takes place, it is radical enough for Jesus to refer to it as a second birth (hence the now overused and misappropriated term "born again") with manifestations in day-to-day living becoming evident with the passage of months and years.

Overall, the Bible contains much more story than doctrine, and is all about relationships rather than religion. Scripture repeatedly describes the bonds between God and ourselves in terms of the loving intimacy of family, similar to those between parent and child, husband and wife (and for the animal lovers, shepherds and sheep). All are appropriate images, and all give great insight. For example, raising children provides a deeper understanding of the extent to which God is willing to love, comfort, educate, exhort, and at times discipline us for our own good. And herein lies an area in which many women, even those who have logged years of time in God's family, need some adjustments.

What sort of adjustments?

Unfortunately, even those who have made a formal commitment to Christ, who understand his death on our behalf, who make the effort to attend church and bring the kids and contribute time and money, will still harbor some bitterness over losses and crosses currently borne. And most hold a few dark secrets which have been carefully guarded and protected through the years. In the mid-life years, these have a way of beginning to clamor for attention, and suddenly spiritual equilibrium becomes a precarious commodity.

During the busy years when we are young, it is relatively easy to ignore those personal issues that we *know*, on some level, must be dealt with some day. But as we begin to slow down, a black cloud from our younger years threatens to overshadow everything, and many women find themselves in a complete malaise during their forties or fifties. We believe this depression is a crisis of the soul wherein a woman is asking the basic question, "Who *am* I?" After twenty-odd years of being everywhere and everything for everybody else, she simply begins to wonder if her existence counts. And whatever past shame lurks in the system begins oozing, unbidden and unwelcome, into the present consciousness.

So there's some housecleaning involved in that famous question "Who am I?"

Absolutely. Perhaps the most important preparation a woman can make for the peri- and postmenopausal years is to clear her accounts with God. One of the most poignant passages in the entire Bible is Psalm 51—a heartrending expression of David's utter regret and longing to be restored to God's favor after his sinful choices surrounding his lust for Bathsheba. "For I know my transgressions, and my sin is always before me.... Create in me a pure heart, O God, and renew a steadfast spirit within me.... Restore to me the joy of your salvation.... A broken and contrite heart, O God, you will not despise."

And the story of the "lost" son in Luke 15 is the perfect illustration of God's response to a contrite heart. After squandering his inheritance, the son comes to his senses and realizes that even the least of his father's servants have a higher standard of living than he is currently enduring. Never dreaming that his father would give him a second chance, he prepares his pathetic speech all the way home. You know the rest of the story: the father is overjoyed that his son has returned home and restores him to his former position in the family.

I have found that, even after I have dealt with my dirty laundry before God, I have a hard time accepting the fact that I can still have a close relationship with him. What's blocking this from happening?

You're not alone. In fact, you're the rule rather than the exception. Why is it so hard for us to grasp how much God longs to be in relationship with us? More often than not, it is because most of us were raised by parents who didn't know how to love us unconditionally. In a perfect world, every child would be raised with this consistent parental message: "You are a miracle. You are an unending marvel and delight to us. We love you—period. When you do something willfully wrong, we will gently correct you until you repent, but it is a pre-established fact that we will always forgive you and get our relationship back on track. How could it be otherwise? *You are our child!*"

But we live in a bent, imperfect world where parents are just doing the best they can, given the kind of parenting *they* survived. Too many children are raised with this kind of message: "I will love you *if* you are good, pretty, compliant, athletic, or smart. If you make too much trouble, if you don't fit into my idea of what a child should be like, I won't love you any more." Our basic sense of self has been derived from the parental messages we received. Sadly, a majority of people hear a conditional message (or something far worse), and then spend the rest of their lives desperately trying to prove that they are worthy of being loved.

The long process of marriage and childrearing gives us an active arena in which we may try to prove our worthiness (or else it keeps us so busy that we have little time to think much about it). But eventually—usually during the mid-life years—we realize we are on a futile quest, because there is no perfect home, no glitchless marriage, no children without problems, no complete financial security, no position or title without hassles, no honors or accolades that don't eventually fade from memory. We are also finally forced to turn around and face the haunting specters of old secrets and feelings of inferiority.

In a way, this universal lack of perfection in our lives serves an extremely valuable purpose—as a gentle (or harsh) reminder that the only true sense of identity and worth comes from our relationship with God. Quite simply, we are worthy only because God assigned worthiness to us, and *not* because we could ever have earned that worthiness. This alone is the basis of a healthy self-concept.

So how do I overcome this glitch in my relationship with God?

At the risk of sounding incredibly trite, make sure you have a regular time and place which is dedicated to the process of getting to know God. Pick up your Bible, dust it off, and make the commitment to spend fifteen to thirty minutes a day listening to the one Being in the universe who loves you perfectly. Too often the notion of a "quiet time" is hamstrung by habits or rituals that do little to build a relationship. Reading the Bible is important—but is it done with thoughtful questions about what God wants say to us, or does it become merely a speed-reading exercise to fulfill this month's "through the Bible in a year" installment? Prayer is important, but is it spoken in stilted seventeenth-century language, or a series of "gimmes," or a message left on God's answering machine? How would your husband or best friend feel if you conversed with him or her that way? Obviously a sense of awe, wonder, and reverence is due to the Creator of the universe, but that doesn't preclude intimacy and honesty.

In addition to a specific time of day that serves as an appointment, much can be accomplished during a literal "running" conversation—while in the car on errands, for example. In fact, talking to God out loud during these times can promote a less disjointed train of thought. (People in the next car may think you're a little psychotic as you appear to talk to yourself in traffic, but that's their problem.) These moments often provide a better opportunity to clear the air about attitude problems, open up various issues, and pray for other people.

In addition to building your relationship with God on your own, conversations with those who are further up the road can be of great value. You might choose a pastor, a support group, or a woman in your church who has a visible track record of her intimacy with God. If you continue to hit roadblocks in this area, especially if you feel they may arise from past hurts or even outright abuse you have suffered in the past, a Christian therapist may be able to help you. Indeed, if you know or believe you have been victimized, even decades ago, it is imperative that you deal with these events under the care of someone who knows how to approach them.

Also, don't forget the wealth of books that offer you the luxury of extended time and repetition to grasp their insights. Our favorites in the area of relating to God are *Knowing God* by J.I. Packer, *Loving God* by Charles Colson, and *The Blessing* by Gary Smalley.

This is not to brag, but what if I've enjoyed a good ongoing relationship with God over the years? Where do I go from here?

Onward and upward! You are in a tremendous position as

you approach and pass through menopause to deepen your intimacy with God and explore new opportunities to serve him. As we will discuss further at the end of this book, there is no limit to the possibilities for you to lend your mind, hands, heart, and wealth of experience to worthwhile projects, both near and far. Your biggest problem, hopefully, will be figuring out how to sort and prioritize the options open to you. You're never too old to get overcommitted, but it's a better problem to deal with than boredom and apathy.

Furthermore, in a culture that has lost its grip on moral values, you are among those who remember the cultural consensus of a few decades ago. Unfortunately, the upcoming generation of "Baby Busters" (loosely defined as those born after 1965) has seen only the current haze of sexual anarchy, media dominated by the morally impaired, and traditional family structures under siege by aggressive social engineers. Those with a Christian perspective, and some godly but incendiary concern over the fate of our nation, can contribute some serious prayer and shoe leather as they join—or, for that matter, lead—those who are standing firm against a malignant tide.

Chapter Five

∽∾∽

Taming Depression, Anxiety, and Other Beasts

Is it my imagination, or does emotional turmoil go hand-in-hand with menopause?

Hand-in-hand is not exactly the right phrase. Some women sail through menopause with relatively little emotional upheaval. Unfortunately, however, most people perceive menopause as an inevitably stormy passage. As we pointed out in Chapter Two, mood problems may accompany declining estrogen levels and usually respond dramatically when estrogen is replaced. This is particularly common when a woman has a track record of mood swings correlating with her monthly cycle prior to menopause.

But menopause does not automatically produce emotional instability, and so moodiness during this time cannot automatically be attributed to hormonal changes. Many factors may stir the emotional waters, including genetics, personal circumstances and conflicts, uncertainty over changing roles, and even spiritual issues. Obviously, no one's life is free from trouble. In fact, in direct contrast to what most of us would desire for ourselves, the apostle James told us to "consider it pure joy" when we encounter various trials because of the growth and learning they eventually can stimulate.

But for some—indeed, more often than you might think—the emotional weather blows hard and cold for prolonged periods of time. It is those persistent and disruptive dips (or plunges) of mood below normal that concern us here.

This may seem like a dumb question, but what are the characteristics of depression?

That's not a dumb question at all, because this problem presents itself in a number of very different ways. In its most extreme form, depression involves an extended experience of intensely negative feelings: sadness, a bleak outlook on the future, and a lack of any joy or pleasure in life, perhaps seasoned with deep regrets or anger. Uncontrollable crying, thoughts that life isn't worth living, and even thoughts of suicide round out this unpleasant picture. Someone in this sort of emotional abyss needs help as soon as possible. Depression more frequently manifests itself with less severe but still doggedly persistent symptoms that often bring people to their family practitioners or internists, rather than to counselors or psychiatrists. Some research has suggested that this problem affects 15 to 30 percent of people visiting medical offices at any given time.

What are the most common symptoms?

By far the most common is fatigue—day in, day out, morning and night, unrelieved by sleep. Usually someone whose primary complaint is chronic tiredness is concerned that some terrible disease is lurking below the surface. But unless there are obvious physical findings suggesting otherwise, less than one in ten will prove to have a specific illness. About half of the rest are actually dealing with depression.

What would lead you to that conclusion?

Usually other symptoms point in that direction. One of the most common is a sleep disturbance: either difficulty falling or staying asleep, a desire to sleep all the time, or insomnia at night and drowsiness all day. Another is a change in appetite: either disinterest in food or just the opposite, with weight soaring either up or down. Concentration may be poor, and little problems and decisions can assume gargantuan proportions. Somewhere along the way, this tired person will also admit to having a prevailing mood which is generally south of neutral, with minor aggravations often provoking a response out of proportion to the annoyance.

And this is depression?

If enough of these symptoms are prevailing, and no other physical cause can account for them, depression is a very likely diagnosis.

But a lot of people have these symptoms.

That's right. And a lot of these people are in fact depressed, even though they may be surprised (or even offended) if their physician broaches this subject. But from a medical perspective, depression encompasses not only overtly unhappy feelings and moods, but an underlying biochemical disturbance in the central nervous system.

What sort of disturbance is that?

Human and animal research, combined with the experience of physicians with millions of patients, has led to the assumption that changes in the level of various neurotransmitters—the chemical compounds that carry messages between cells in the brain—cause specific physical and emotional symptoms.

What would cause a change in neurotransmitter levels?

This usually involves a complex interplay of genetics and circumstances. The genetic component is often revealed when close relatives display the same symptoms, although those who are a generation removed may have attributed them to "nerves" or simply suffered in silence. The genetic predisposition may lead to a depressive episode that is being triggered by a stressful event, but it may also come literally "out of the blue." A person may be unable to pin down a specific problem or issue which has set the symptoms in motion, leading to the conclusion that they must be "going crazy" because they feel so lousy without any provocation. (By the way, it's a good rule of thumb that if you are worried about being crazy, you're not. Genuinely psychotic people rarely can be convinced that there is anything wrong with their bizarre, derailed trains of thought.)

Is there any way to measure what the neurotransmitters are doing?

Unfortunately, not at this time. No blood test, X-ray, MRI scan or other technology tells the tale as well as a person's history and list of complaints.

Are you saying that every depression is basically a biochemical problem? If so, that would be a convenient way to avoid a lot of personal responsibility.

Good point. Think of the depressive episode as a river fed by a number of streams. In some cases the problem is primarily biochemical, very often with a laundry list of physical symptoms dominating the picture. In others, the depression is a direct outgrowth of the issues of life: past hurts or overt abuse, conflicts in important relationships, situational stressors, and spiritual problems. A significant event or an ongoing issue can also trigger a biochemical deficiency. In the majority of situations, there is a mixed bag of biochemistry and problems of living, all of which need to be addressed.

What can be done about the neurotransmitters if they appear to be a major part of the problem?

A variety of medications, known collectively as antidepressants (what a surprise...), can be extremely helpful. Contrary to a common misperception, these are not "happy pills." They do not induce a state of bliss but restore mood to a neutral level. They are not physically addicting or psychologically habit forming. None are controlled substances, and no one sells them on the street.

For years the so-called tricyclic antidepressants were virtually the only game in town. They are still useful today, although their side effects are legendary: dry mouth, blurry vision, constipation, and occasionally faintness. Furthermore, in an overdose—not a trivial risk in someone who is seriously depressed—they can produce some dicey situations with heart rhythm, among other things.

Over the past few years, the medical treatment of depression has improved drastically with the development of newer agents with fewer side effects and greater safety. These include Prozac®, Zoloft®, Paxil®, and Wellbutrin®.

Wait a minute. I've heard that Prozac® is really dangerous and causes people to act crazy or suicidal.

Prozac® has gotten some bad press, much of which can be attributed to one particular organization. But two thorough reviews of this drug by the Food and Drug Administration have failed to demonstrate that Prozac® is associated with any more problems than anything else on the market. Nevertheless, the rumors still circulate, and some vague uneasiness about this drug persists.

Are there any specific problems with these newer drugs?

Compared to the tricyclics, adverse reactions to Prozac® and the others tend to be unpredictable and infrequent. Individuals have reported feeling sedated or "hyper," headaches, stomach upsets, and a vague collection of sensory disturbances, but not on a wide scale. Actually, the most common problem is simply a failure to produce any obvious change.

What happens in a best case scenario?

When things work well, the antidepressant parts the emotional clouds and gradually brings physical functioning and emotions back to a normal, neutral level. "I feel like my old self" is a common expression of improvement. One woman aptly described it as the difference between believing her menopause symptoms were the harbinger of old age and the ability to exclaim, "Thank you, God, that this is just a hot flash and not a terminal illness—a hot flash I can deal with!"

The key word is *gradual*. These medications are not a quick fix, and a certain amount of trial and error may be necessary before finding the right drug and dose. In fact, while some symptoms such as insomnia typically improve within a week, the better part of a month may pass before all of the benefits are seen.

Once there is some improvement, do you stop the drug?

No. Unlike treating a strep throat with penicillin, treatment for depression should continue for six to twelve months, and often much longer. But because antidepressants are not habit forming, discontinuation is never difficult.

I'm not sure I would be comfortable taking a drug to improve depression. Wouldn't it be better to try to work things out by myself or in counseling first?

That decision should be made with your doctor and counselor. If unresolved issues of life are indeed generating the depression, medications will make little or no difference (or at most produce a few side effects). In such cases, counseling, prayer, input from family and friends, and even loving confrontation may all be necessary for recovery. Destructive habits may need to change, and in almost every case exercise will help.

But it is critical that no potential contributor to a depression be ignored. If a neurotransmitter problem remains untreated, the wisest counsel and the hardest work on issues will bring about progress at a snail's pace or slower. In such cases, taking medication should be considered as appropriate as taking a thyroid supplement if that gland fails to function adequately, or using insulin to treat diabetes if the pancreas no longer supplies it. Any work on issues and relationships will be much more productive when one isn't exhausted or an emotional wreck.

I've heard some pastors and speakers on the radio say that emotional problems are really spiritual issues, and in many ways that makes sense to me. Could taking medication short-circuit what should be done in prayer?

It could theoretically, but the two activities are not mutually exclusive. A biochemical contribution to depression has the same spiritual implications as any other *medical* issue. Seeking healing from God is absolutely appropriate, as it is with pneumonia, heart disease, or any physical disorder—but so is the judicious use of tools which can help restore a normal, productive life.

There can be, on the other hand, spiritual roots to depression which no medication can touch. Estrangement from God, especially when it is prolonged, will not contribute to healthy and stable emotions. Many depressions stem from prolonged anger and bitterness, which ultimately turn inward like a malignant drill into the soul. The Bible's frequent insistence that we be willing to forgive others for their transgressions against us isn't merely a theological nicety. The act of forgiveness, rather than being some artificial effort to "feel good" about someone who has harmed us, really represents our giving up the right to seek revenge and harbor bitterness. It is to be done for our own healing.

In some situations, a depression can actually occur in the wake of a major personal or spiritual battle, even when the result is a victory. One of the best examples of this type of "crash" is the aftermath of Elijah's conflict with the prophets of Baal. After presiding over a resounding demonstration of God's superiority over a false deity, Elijah literally fell apart. He fled in terror from the hostile Queen Jezebel and finally collapsed in exhaustion under a tree. "I have had enough, Lord," he sighed. "Take my life" (1 Kgs 19:4). After some nourishment and conversation with God, this episode passed.

Our point in this chapter is that emotional turmoil may have spiritual, relational, historical, or physical roots. None of them should be ignored.

Speaking of turmoil, doesn't anxiety fit right into this discussion?

It does, indeed, and much of what has already been said applies to this very common disturbance. In fact, in many cases anxiety is actually a component of depression, and it responds to the same treatments. However, the medical treatment for anxiety, in contrast to depression, consists almost entirely of symptom control rather than cure. Furthermore, the most immediately effective and commonly used medications, the benzodiazepenes, are all habit forming. If given regularly for more than a week or two, they must be weaned carefully to avoid withdrawal reactions.

In the midst of a sudden and severe crisis, these medications can be extremely useful. For example, in the aftermath of the January, 1994 Northridge, California earthquake (which hit us as we were finishing this book!), many people began to experience uncontrollable fear, chest pains, shortness of breath, and palpitations whenever a sizable aftershock rumbled across the city. Most of this was aggravated by lack of sleep, and much of it was drastically improved by judicious short-term doses of benzodiazepene medications such as Xanax® and Ativan®.

What about long-term anxiety?

This is another story altogether. Some clinicians feel that this is caused by a biochemical problem in the brain, as has been postulated with depression. This notion gains some credibility when we deal with people who feel anxious and suffer multitudes of associated physical symptoms, despite years of therapy, prayer, and medical reassurance. Try as they might, they simply cannot achieve any sense of equilibrium (let alone relaxation) without some sort of medication.

On the other hand, very often someone with a history of chronic anxiety has yet to deal with some important issues from the past, often involving abuse and neglect. When a child's trust and vulnerability are violated by one or more adults, or if basic needs for love and security are ignored (or replaced by insults), the consequences play out for years. We have dealt with victims of childhood abuse who live in a state of never-ending "red alert," who see the world as a perpetually dangerous and hostile place. This continuous discomfort and hypervigilance must be relieved eventually, and all too often drugs (prescription or street) serve that purpose—for years on end.

While there certainly can be a place for the judicious use of medication to help the traumatized person function more normally, the most far-reaching results are to be found through counseling with someone who can deal with the past hurts and bring God into the picture as a very real, perfect parent.

Does the arrival of menopause create more difficulty for someone with this problem?

It certainly may, depending on a host of factors. If a woman has compensated for past hurts and insecurities by using beauty or sexuality as a form of empowerment, the gradual loss of those attributes can be frightening indeed. If a woman has derived her identity from childrearing, as we discussed in the last chapter, the ending of her reproductive years may also seem to signal the literal end of her purpose and meaning.

If some health problems accompany the postmenopausal years, fear of doctors, disability, and death may cause considerable agitation—which may in turn aggravate the illness or generate a carload of confusing symptoms.

What kind of symptoms?

No strong emotional event occurs without some physiological responses. The degree of response may vary, as will the part of the anatomy which feels it most acutely. Anxiety can generate a rapid, pounding pulse; a sensation of tightening in the chest; shortness of breath, which can lead to hyperventilation in a futile effort to "get enough air"; headaches; acid indigestion; and cramping throughout the intestinal tract, especially in the colon. And these are just the common symptoms. Chronically anxious people are sometimes beset with migratory aches and pains, strange patterns of numbness and tingling, and vague sensations that "something isn't right" in the head or elsewhere.

What can be done about these?

If a woman with symptoms such as these has not already made a number of visits to her doctor or the emergency room (out of a justifiable concern that something serious is going on in the heart, lungs, or other vital organs), she should sit down with her physician, run through her list of symptoms, and put up with whatever tests are necessary to investigate them. If the verdict is that no dire illness is in progress and that anxiety or depression may be involved, this should be accepted with some thanksgiving.

Why is that?

Because dealing directly with anxiety is ultimately better than confronting a serious medical problem.

Then what?

Get to work on the issues. Spiritually, it is critical to become thoroughly convinced of God's care, provision, and faithfulness. Jesus had a great deal to say about anxiety, about our inability to add a cubit to our life span by worrying. His words need to be taken seriously. Some prayerful, practical work with a counselor, support group, or (better yet) both is in order to identify the past and current sources of pain and fear. If you don't notice immediate improvement, remember that neither Rome nor your response patterns to life were built in a day. But never take your eyes off the ultimate goal of renewing your mind, of revamping its responses to life's curve balls and left turns. The apostle Paul stated so eloquently in his letter to the Roman believers:

> Do not conform any longer to the pattern of this world, but be transformed by the renewing of your mind. Then you will be able to test and approve what God's will is—his good, pleasing and perfect will. Rom 12:2.

God wants us to be free from the chains of anxiety, turmoil, and depression so that we may love God with all our heart, soul, mind, and strength. Difficult emotional issues are not resolved instantly, but they *can* be resolved. Medical issues can be treated and stabilized or even cured. If you struggle with these areas, seek the assistance you need so that you can discover how exciting and fulfilling your life can be.

Chapter Six

ⷜⷜ

The "E" Word:
Should I Use Estrogen?

It seems that whenever menopause is mentioned, the words "hormone supplement" nearly always follow on the next breath. Is estrogen merely a cultural fad, or is it a genuine source of benefit?

Over the past three decades, the status of hormone replacement therapy—which we will abbreviate HRT from here on—has swung wildly, both in the general public and among medical professionals. In the 1950s the successes of estrogen in relieving acute symptoms (such as hot flashes), vaginal atrophy, and (for some) mood swings led to a naive, "wonder drug" mentality. Estrogen seemed to be good for "whatever ails ya" if you were female and over forty, and by the early 1960s it was the fifth most commonly written prescription in the United States.

Then in the mid-1970s a new series of studies showed that long-term estrogen users were at a higher risk for developing cancer of the uterus. As other concerns were raised about links between estrogen and breast cancer, blood clots, and other problems, the general perception of HRT changed from that of a panacea to a rather drastic and risky intervention for those with severe menopausal difficulties.

Meanwhile, a great deal of experience and research over the next twenty years has both refined HRT and shown some important long-range benefits. But until recently these advantages have not been as widely known (or believed) in the general population. As a result, even with more coverage now showing up in the popular media, only about 15 percent of post menopausal women in the United States who could potentially benefit from HRT actually use it.

So what kinds of problems does estrogen help solve?

We would like to divide estrogen's potential targets into *symptom problems*, which are merely annoying, and *silent problems*, which are dangerous.

The symptoms that estrogen can improve were detailed in Chapter Two. But for a quick recap, they are:

1. The infamous hot flashes and flushes.
2. Night sweats if they are caused by declining estrogen levels.
3. Vaginal atrophy, and its associated irritation, itching, and burning.
4. Urinary tract symptoms such as incontinence, frequency, and burning, if they are caused by low-estrogen atrophy.
5. Formication, the sensation that insects are crawling on the skin.
6. Aging and wrinkling of skin, to some degree. Estrogen does not reverse the effects of an abundance of birthdays, sun exposure, and cigarette smoking on skin, but most authorities believe that thinning and wrinkling develops more slowly with hormone replacement.
7. Emotional instability and irritability in some (but certainly not all) women. This must be evaluated, like virtually

every item on this list, on a case-by-case basis.

Estrogen supplementation, whether on a short or long-term basis, can provide significant relief for these symptoms. We'll address some general questions about the use of estrogen later.

But first let's deal with two very important medical issues which frequently respond favorably to HRT: osteoporosis and cardiovascular disease. Both conditions are major concerns for women at mid-life and beyond—and both are silent, until it's too late.

ESTROGEN AND OSTEOPOROSIS

You've mentioned it several times. But what exactly is osteoporosis?

Osteoporosis, which literally means "porous bone," is a condition in which bone mass is gradually lost, resulting in less strength and an increased risk of fractures.

And this is pretty common?

Very common: twenty million Americans are affected, according to current estimates.

What are the results for those twenty million?

Thin, porous bones break easily, often with very slight or even no trauma. Simply shifting position or bending over can provoke a fracture—often of the leg or hip, and in some severe cases, of the spine. Over 1.5 million fractures caused by osteoporosis occur every year in the United States. Of these, 250,000 involve the hip, generating an amazing $10 billion annual bill for acute and long-term care. But more ominous is the fact that 15 to 20 percent of those who suffer a broken hip will die within a year after the fracture. Thousands of other people suffer painful fractures of the vertebra and forearm every year. And gradual compressing of the weight-bearing segments of the spine eventually leads to the deforming curvatures—especially the impolitely-named "dowager's hump"—which bother so many elderly women.

As our population continues to age, the annual number of fractures will double within forty years unless some meaningful preventive measures are taken by many people—primarily perimenopausal women.

How does osteoporosis happen?

Contrary to a common perception that the skeleton is lifeless, bone is living tissue. At any given time, various areas are undergoing turnover and remodeling, which blends microscopic resorption (tearing down) and rebuilding processes. These normally are tightly coupled to one another, but any imbalance between them will lead to a net gain or loss of bone.

Unfortunately, after reaching a peak between age thirty and thirty-five, the bone mass of both men and women begins a steady and relentless decline with age. The speed of loss over time, and its impact, are determined by several factors.

1. Gender. The peak bone mass reached in early adulthood is about 30 percent more in men than in women.

2. Race. Black women tend to have a greater bone density than white or Asian women, and are less commonly affected by osteoporosis.

3. Age. Between the ages of fifty and eighty, a woman loses *30 percent* of her bone density. During the first five years after menopause, the loss is fastest—about 2 percent per year, after which the rate drops to 1 percent per year. It stands to reason that the oldest women have the thinnest bones and thus the most fractures. Half of all hip fractures occur after age eighty.

4. Early menopause. As soon as the ovaries retire, or if they are surgically removed, the accelerated bone loss begins. Some recent research suggests that it is the *total number of reproductive years* (that is, the age at menopause minus the age of the first menstrual period) that makes the difference. Women with thirty or fewer reproductive years tend to have significantly lower bone mineral density than their counterparts with forty or more reproductive years. Thus a late start and early end of cycles does not bode well for strong bones.

So estrogen has something to do with this?

Absolutely. When estrogen levels drop, the balance in bone remodeling is lost: the cells that rebuild bone (called *osteoblasts*) slow down, while those that tear it down (called *osteoclasts*) pick up steam. And the longer estrogen levels are low, the more bone you lose.

So taking estrogen can prevent bone loss?

Right, but we'll get to that in a minute. Moving on to the other risk factors for osteoporosis:

5. Thin body build. Osteoporosis is about the only health problem for which being heavy is a theoretical advantage. Higher weight leads to a greater peak in bone mass when young, more production of estrogen (in fatty tissue) after menopause, and increased bone formation stimulated by weight-bearing forces throughout life. These advantages, of course, are greatly offset by other risks when the scale reads too high.

6. Sedentary lifestyle. As just mentioned, bones that support weight are stimulated to preserve their density by muscles pulling and moving them. Whether from prolonged immobility (from chronic illness or while recuperating from an injury) or a lifestyle devoid of exercise, the same problem occurs over time.

7. Smoking. In addition to their obscenely long list of other health risks, cigarettes contribute to osteoporosis both before and after menopause. This is probably caused by an anti-estrogen effect of nicotine.

8. Alcohol. Medical truism: the relationship between alcohol consumption and bone mass before menopause is both inverse and dose-dependent. English translation: the more you drink, and the longer you drink it, the thinner your bones will be.

9. Low calcium intake. Of all the dietary factors studied by osteoporosis researchers, calcium (in food or supplement) has been found to make the most important contribution to bone strength throughout life.

10. Certain medications. Oral cortisone preparations, such as might be used to treat chronic bronchitis, asthma, or severe arthritis, definitely accelerate bone loss. For most long-term lung problems which need cortisone, the medication can be inhaled (with far less absorption into the rest of the body). But some people with rheumatoid arthritis, lupus, and related disorders may need cortisone to control their symptoms, although physicians invariably try to use alternative approaches. Anyone on long-term oral cortisone should take special precautions to protect against excessive bone loss.

So if I am a thin, aging, white or Asian, smoking, drinking, milk-hating, cortisone-taking couch potato, I may need an orthopedist in the future?

Correct. Keep your health insurance premiums paid up, and try to avoid tripping over anything. A better approach, of course, would be to take some preventive action.

And what might that be, as if I couldn't guess?

You can't change your age, sex, race, body build, or (usually) the timing of menopause, so you're off the hook on those counts. But if you are at higher risk, you need to pay close attention to the other risk factors that you *can* change. As for smoking, alcohol, and exercise, take yet another look at the "Basic Maintenance Checklist" in Chapter Three.

To prevent osteoporosis, exercise should be *weight bearing* if at all possible. That is, feet are making contact with the ground and bones are supporting the body. This, and to some degree muscle building exercise as well, causes very slight distortion of bone, which in turn stimulates the bone to build more supportive tissue. The best all around exercise, also noted in Chapter Three, is a basic walking program (with appropriate warm-up stretching and cool-down). Walking is simple, cheap, low-risk, and helpful to heart and lung functions as well.

The other key preventive measures are adequate calcium on a daily basis, and supplemental estrogen.

How much calcium are we talking about?

The National Institutes of Health and other august bodies have for some time recommended that women routinely consume one thousand mg. of calcium per day before menopause, and fifteen hundred mg. after. Since a typical daily intake of calcium from diet in the United States provides about four hundred to five hundred mg., some sort of supplementation is usually a good idea.

What sorts of foods supply the most calcium?

As you have probably heard through the media grapevine, dairy products have a decided edge in the calcium supply. A one-cup (eight-ounce) glass of *any* form of milk (anything between whole and skim) contains about three hundred mg. of calcium, so consuming a quart per day (or four of these servings) approaches twelve hundred mg., and thus provides nearly the entire recommended daily amount for a post-menopausal woman. An eight-ounce serving of low-fat plain yogurt contains more than four hundred mg. of calcium. Salmon and sardines are also heavy hitters: three ounces of these provides about 160 mg. and 370 mg. respectively.

Obviously, a concern with any of these items might be the fat and calorie content, but the numbers actually aren't too bad. Skim milk, for example, contains 90 calories per eight ounces, or 360 per quart. One percent milk, which most of us find much more palatable, contains only 15 more calories per eight ounces than nonfat (105 vs. 90 calories), or 420 per quart. Obviously, for those who need to restrict calories to maintain or lose weight, this is a healthy chunk of the total.

You got that right. What about foods not derived from animals?

Leafy green vegetables such as collards, kale, and turnip greens—obviously a hot item in most diets—are respectable calcium sources. The more common greens in a small salad provide about 100 mg., an orange or a half cup of raisins about 50 mg., and a half dozen figs about 150 mg. And some vegetables such as spinach and Swiss chard contain oxalic acid, which may block some calcium absorption.

I think I fall in that 500 mg. per day calcium diet zone. Should I be taking supplements?

This would be a good idea, since it's possible to make up the difference without taking much out of your pocketbook. Fortunately, you don't need some fancy formulation to get the job done.

I notice that there's no shortage of brands at the store. How do I decide what to use?

Calcium is always attached to another compound, the character of which may affect absorption and overall cost. The most commonly used and most cost-effective preparations use calcium carbonate, the active ingredient in many chewable antacids. (Tums E-X®, for example, contains 300 mg. per tablet, so four of these per day provides a very respectable supplement for about fifteen cents.) Absorption is usually enhanced by taking these with food, and the total amount should not be consumed in one sitting, but divided into two or three doses. Obviously, if you are already consuming a pint or more of milk per day, your intake should be adjusted accordingly.

Some people feel bloated or otherwise distressed with calcium carbonate and may want to consider alternatives such as calcium gluconate, lactate, or citrate. Of these, calcium citrate is considered to be particularly well-absorbed, but it may require several tablets per day to reach recommended doses.

If 1,500 mg. of calcium per day is a good idea, would I get even more benefit from doubling that amount?

Loading up on higher than recommended doses of *anything* is rarely a good idea, and calcium is no exception. Doses that far exceed the 1,500 mg. level may increase your risk for kidney stones or actually raise your blood concentration of calcium, which is normally tightly regulated.

What about Vitamin D?

Again, the key word is moderation. A daily intake of 400 IU is adequate to promote absorption of calcium. Vitamin D is actually hard to avoid, since it is usually added to milk, vitamin fortified cereals, multi-vitamin tablets, and many calcium supplements. Deliberately taking large doses of Vitamin D (surpassing 1,000 IU per day), unless under supervision for a specific medical reason, can cause calcium to be *removed* from bone.

Do exercise and adequate calcium intake by themselves provide enough protection from bone loss, or do I need to do more?

If you are consistent in these two measures for years on end, you will be way ahead of the pack. Keep it up! However, most of the current literature indicates that for most women bone loss continues (though at a lesser rate) after menopause, even when one is doing all the right things, because of the important role of estrogen in bone metabolism.

So hormone replacement therapy is a good idea, even when the other bone-preserving activities are going on?

The medical literature has consistently demonstrated that of all the preventive measures designed to preserve bone mass, estrogen replacement is the most effective. It will, in fact, enhance the effects of the other approaches. Furthermore, the benefit is the greatest when started soon after menopause (within the first few years, and preferably right away), and continues as long as the supplementation is given.

So it doesn't work to take estrogen for those first few years when the bone loss is the fastest, and then quit?

It will help for those few years, but as soon as the supplement stops the bone loss starts.

So you're talking about long-term use of estrogen for this problem?

Right—at least until age seventy-five, and arguably for the rest of a woman's life. Despite what has been suggested in the past, even most "late starters" (for whom five or more unsupplemented years have elapsed since menopause) will derive some benefit from HRT as well.

And you're talking about estrogen being the rule rather than the exception?

Because of the magnitude of the suffering and costs generated by osteoporosis, the pendulum is swinging now toward asking who *shouldn't* receive HRT rather than who should. Some literature suggests that estrogen replacement started at menopause and continued indefinitely cuts a woman's ultimate risk of a hip fracture in half.

ESTROGEN AND CARDIOVASCULAR DISEASE

You said a little earlier that taking estrogen can reduce the risk of heart disease. How much do women approaching menopause need to be concerned about the health of their heart?

All women need to become "heart smart" if they want to "live long and prosper" (to quote Mr. Spock). Far more women die from cardiovascular (heart and blood vessel) disease than from all forms of cancer *combined*. Coronary heart disease (CHD) in particular kills 250,000 women every year in the United States. That represents one out of three female deaths, an ominous ratio. (By comparison, less than 3 percent of women will die from breast cancer, and less than 1 percent from ovarian cancer.) So while it's important to mind the cancer store by having PAP smears, breast checks, mammograms, sigmoidoscopies, and other indignities at their appointed times, failing to pay attention to the heart could prove to be a lethal oversight.

What is coronary disease, anyway?

The coronary arteries provide a constant and critical supply of blood (and thus oxygen) to heart muscle. (Their name is derived from "corona" or crown, suggested by their configuration around the upper half of the heart.) Unfortunately, they have a tendency to become choked and clogged by fatty plaques, as we discussed earlier.

When the body needs to do any amount of work beyond total rest, the demands on the heart and its blood supply immediately increase. But if the heart muscle needs more blood than can flow through the narrowed coronaries, pain may develop (called *angina*), or a full blown heart attack (a dumb but enduring term for the death of any portion of heart muscle). In medicalese this event is called a *myocardial infarction,* or MI. As the muscle dies, it becomes more "twitchy" and irritable, which can cause a life-threatening rhythm change. Or it may leave the heart with less muscle-power to do its daily work, somewhat like a car whose engine has lost a cylinder or two. This can result in a maddening and at times overwhelming mix of symptoms, including loss of stamina, shortness of breath (caused by accumulation of fluid in the lungs), and swelling of the legs.

It sounds like coronary artery disease is something to be avoided at all costs. But isn't it really a "guy thing"?

Only in the sense that it shows up sooner in men. But by ten years after menopause, the disease and death rates from CHD in women catch up to those observed in men. And once the problem shows up, it is actually *more* lethal in women.

Looking from another direction: one in seven women between the ages of forty-five and sixty-four has some form of CHD. After age sixty-five, that number is one in *three*. And, alas, two out of three women who are afflicted with CHD will die from it.

And how exactly does CHD show itself?

In 20 percent of people (either gender), the first symptom is dropping dead. No warning, no chance to talk to the doctor, no saying good-bye to loved ones, no tying up of loose ends—just a very sudden departure from this life. Another 50 percent of people with CHD have an MI—the killing of some heart muscle, and all of its consequences, including a vacation in the hospital—as their first event. Only 30 percent get any advance notice in the form of angina, the reversible, usually attention-grabbing chest pain.

So it's better to try to prevent CHD rather than wait for symptoms to show up?

Definitely, absolutely, seriously better.

And prevention consists of...?

Just like with osteoporosis: modifying the risk factors you can do something about. You can't change your age or your pedigree. Unfortunately, if any of your parents or siblings have had CHD (especially early in life), you probably are at higher risk. But you *can* do the following:

1. Quit smoking. There are multitudes of compelling reasons to kick tobacco out of your life, but this is one of the biggest. Four out of ten coronary disease deaths are directly related to the burning butts, and premenopausal smokers carry three times the risk of an MI compared to their nonpolluting counterparts.

2. Keep your blood pressure under control. (And if you don't know what it is, find out.) The "Basic Maintenance Checklist" in Chapter Three reviewed the various lifestyle and medical strategies for bringing the pressure under control. But if you have other risk factors, you may need to consider medication more seriously, in order to gain control sooner rather than later.

3. Lower your cholesterol—especially the LDL portion— and your triglycerides. And try to raise your HDL while you're at it. If you've forgotten what you learned in your cholesterol drills, review Chapter Three. The test will come later....

4. Check your glucose (blood sugar) level. If it is elevated, work with your doctor to bring it down. If you know you have diabetes, keep your glucose as low as possible (without driving it below normal levels). Persistent high blood glucose levels increase your risk for CHD and accelerate its progress. In fact, the presence of diabetes in women before menopause negates their gender advantage over men in the same age group.

The management of diabetes is well beyond the scope of this book, but we should note that 80 percent of cases develop later in life, and in the majority of cases the glucose can be controlled by adhering to our familiar advice: shedding excess pounds, maintaining regular exercise, and favoring complex carbohydrates over simple sugars and fats.

5. Get off the couch and start some aerobic exercise. If you have an excellent memory, you may recall from Chapter Three that exercise increases the level of HDL, the "good" cholesterol. And you may also recall that even modest levels of exercise—a half-hour walk four times per week—significantly reduces CHD risk.

6. Seriously consider long-term hormone replacement therapy. Estimates vary, but the overall trend of research points to a 30 to 50 percent reduction in the risk for CHD and its complications (including death) for long-term estrogen users. The higher number is likely the more accurate estimate.

How does estrogen protect the heart?

One significant effect appears to be on lipids: estrogen use appears to lower the LDL ("bad") cholesterol and raise the HDL ("good") cholesterol components. The amount of change will depend on the starting level, the particular form used, the dose, and so forth. Estrogen also seems to have a direct effect on the formation of plaque in the arteries. Furthermore, it probably dilates coronary arteries, which increases blood flow through them.

Some research suggests that estrogen given by patch (Estraderm®) does not improve HDL and LDL levels as much as oral forms. But on the other hand, oral estrogens tend to increase triglyceride levels, which the patch does not change. Knowing your lipid status may therefore have some bearing on the best type of estrogen to use.

I've heard that progesterone, which is given to many women along with estrogen, may increase the risk of coronary disease (and negate the benefit from estrogen).

Adding progesterone during part or all of the monthly cycle, which is almost universal if a woman still has her uterus, may reduce the improvement in HDL brought about by estrogen. But several long-term studies don't show much of a difference when compared to women who take estrogen alone.

So what's the bottom line?

While researchers will continue to fine-tune their conclusions about which form of estrogen does what, there is little doubt that prevention of coronary artery disease is one of the most compelling reasons for taking estrogen on a long-term basis after menopause.

What if I don't have any obvious risk factors for coronary disease? Should I still think about estrogen anyway?

Some women have absolutely no family history of coronary disease, no extra fat, very low cholesterol levels, an active exercise program, and a tobacco-free life. For such women, preventing coronary disease is not going to be high on the list of reasons for using estrogen. But there are other good reasons, especially prevention of osteoporosis, to consider using it after menopause.

You've given a lot of reasons for a woman to consider using hormone replacement therapy after menopause. What are some reasons not to use it.

Before we begin looking at prohibitions, warnings, precautions, and other downsides of estrogen supplementation, keep in mind that the vast majority of women who still have a uterus will be using progesterone along with estrogen as part of the HRT package. Most of the warnings apply to both hormones.

1. HRT should not be used if you are pregnant. There are some potential risks to the developing fetus, especially during early pregnancy.

2. HRT should not be used if you have an undiagnosed breast lump. While it is not likely that estrogen will cause a breast cancer to start (see below), it may stimulate the growth of certain breast tumors. You must find out what is going on before considering using HRT.

3. HRT should not be used if you have abnormal vaginal bleeding which has not been evaluated. As with breast lumps, you also need to know what is happening in this part of your body before adding hormones to the mix. If you have definitely completed your menopause (that is, a year has passed since your last cycle, or the diagnosis has been confirmed by a doctor's exam and lab studies) and you start bleeding again, look out. The lining of the uterus needs to be evaluated for abnormalities, including the possibility of cancer.

4. HRT should be used with extreme caution if you have a history of problems with abnormal blood clotting. If you have ever been treated for a blood clot in the veins of the leg, or a pulmonary embolus (in which a clot travels from a vein in the leg or pelvis to the lung), HRT might increase your risk of a repeat performance. This concern, we should note, is actually based on adverse experiences with the earliest oral contraceptives, which contained very large doses of synthetic estrogen and progesterone. Contraceptives in use today contain much smaller amounts of these compounds, and the hormones used in HRT are in turn far less potent than those in contraceptives. The concern is thus a form of "guilt by association," but it should be reviewed with your physician.

5. HRT should be used with caution if you have liver disease. Again, this is an issue related to the effects of the high-dose oral contraceptives of bygone days. But because estrogen has provoked jaundice in very rare cases, those who already are dealing with an ongoing liver problem should review this situation with an internist or gastroenterologist before beginning HRT. Estrogen also may slightly increase the risk of developing gallstones, but this risk can be offset by losing any excess weight and lowering blood cholesterol levels.

What about the risk of developing cancer of the uterus while on HRT?

For women who take estrogen by itself, the most well-documented cancer risk is of the uterus lining (endometrium). The overall risk for a woman developing this cancer is about 1 in 1,000, and this number increases four- to eight-fold when estrogen is added. This, indeed, is the reason why progesterone is included in nearly every woman's hormone regime if she still has a uterus.

Progesterone, as you may recall from Chapter Two, rounds out the development of this lining every month during the reproductive years. After menopause, it prevents ongoing stimulation of the lining which might induce precancerous changes. In fact, women who use appropriate progesterone doses every month appear to have *less* risk of endometrial cancer than those who don't take anything at all.

Should I be concerned about developing breast cancer as a result of using HRT?

This is by far the biggest worry of women who are considering hormone replacement. So far, more than fifty studies have looked at this issue, and a few "meta-analyses" have combined the results of several studies in order to look for general trends. Some studies have shown an increased risk in certain groups of women, while others have shown a decreased risk (sometimes in the same subgroup). But when the total population studied thus far is considered as a whole, there appears to be no overall change in risk at all. Interestingly, women who develop breast cancer while on HRT have a significantly better life expectancy than those who develop it without hormone replacement.

Why would that be?

Probably because of earlier detection. Women receiving HRT will usually be required to have annual pap smears and breast checks in order to continue their refills. Those without a specific prompting to show up regularly for these chores may let them go, unless they are otherwise compulsive about unpleasant necessities.

Keep in mind also that the risks of developing and dying from cardiovascular disease are immensely greater than those of having breast or uterine cancer, with or without HRT.

Are there any other drawbacks to using HRT?

Some women have side effects from one or both hormones, which may give them second thoughts about years of ongoing use. Dealing with these will involve some individualized decisions about the severity of the side effect compared to the problems HRT is treating. The more common side effects and hassles include:

1. Fluid retention, which can be provoked by either hor-

mone. This may manifest as swelling of hands, feet, or breasts. In some cases, headaches may be provoked, or established patterns worsened. Women who dealt with tender lumps in their breasts every month during their reproductive years may not be thrilled with a series of encores. This may be treated by adjusting the type or dosage of hormone, or in rare instances using a mild diuretic for all or part of the month. Breast tenderness can also be reduced by avoiding caffeine and chocolate.

2. Elevated blood pressure, which may in fact be related to fluid retention.

3. Some irritability (specifically PMS-like symptoms) while taking progesterone.

4. Spotting, or outright vaginal bleeding, which will depend greatly on the pattern of HRT used.

5. Costs of medications and physician consultations. Keep in mind, however, that nearly all of the screening done in connection with using HRT should be done routinely anyway.

If I decide to use hormone replacement therapy, what type should I get?

First of all, before even considering one or another version of HRT, you will need to go over your history and have an appropriate physical exam. Your physician may need to confirm that you are postmenopausal, review risk factors for various problems, screen for breast and cervical cancer, and arrange follow up. You should have time to discuss the pros and cons of HRT for you as an individual (not just as a statistic), and have any questions answered.

Assuming you agree to proceed, you may use one of several

options. A common approach is to create a monthly cycle which is a crude approximation of the premenstrual hormone flow. Estrogen may be given for the first twenty-five days of a calendar month, with progesterone added for the final ten to thirteen days of those twenty-five. During the final five or six days of the month, when no hormones are given, a withdrawal bleed may occur.

That sounds terrible! One of the few things I was looking forward to after menopause was the end of that bleeding hassle. Is there any way to avoid it?

Many women, indeed, don't care to continue the monthly flow. And some find that symptoms of falling estrogen levels come roaring back during the final days of the month. For the latter, estrogen can be continued through the entire month, and the progesterone given at the same time or some other. (Many women prefer to add the progesterone at the beginning of the calendar month, so that they don't have to deal with bleeding at Thanksgiving and the Christmas/New Year's week.)

For those who want to avoid the monthly bleeding altogether, an alternative is to take both estrogen and a smaller dose of progesterone every day of the month. The downside of this approach is the likelihood of some unpredictable spotting, but this usually disappears after a few months.

What if I have had a hysterectomy?

Most women without a uterus will take only the estrogen, since the primary function of the progesterone in HRT (at least thus far) is to protect the uterine lining from overstimulation and reduce the risk of cancer. Obviously, that risk is nonexistent if the uterus is gone. Some researchers have suggested that progesterone may confer some added protection against osteoporosis, but this has not yet translated into widespread use in women who have had a hysterectomy.

What form of estrogen and progesterone should I use?

The vast majority of women using HRT take their hormones orally. Some women, however, do not absorb estrogen as well as others and find the transdermal patch (Estraderm®) more effective. Since this form of estrogen also bypasses the liver, it may hold an advantage for women with liver disease. The patch can be applied to any area of skin (usually on the trunk) and is changed every three and one half days. Progesterone is added during the cycle in one of the ways we have described. One common annoyance is the development of a skin sensitivity, which leaves a rash whenever the patch is removed.

Some women wish only to be relieved of vaginal itching and burning, and they will use one of the estrogen vaginal creams instead of an oral form. This does work locally, but some of the hormone is absorbed as well. Unfortunately, this absorption is of little value: it is not enough to protect against problems such as osteoporosis, but it is too much for the woman who for whatever reason is not supposed to take oral estrogen.

Over the years some women have received their HRT in the form of monthly injections. Because of unpredictable blood levels over a month's time, these have fallen out of favor, except in those very rare circumstances when a woman cannot tolerate oral or transdermal forms.

Is one particular type or brand of hormone more useful than the others?

All of the estrogens in common use for postmenopausal HRT in the United States are referred to as "natural," because they duplicate those forms of estrogen manufactured in the human body. (Synthetic estrogens, on the other hand, are much more potent and utilized in oral contraceptives, whose purpose is to suppress the signals from the brain to the ovaries and thus prevent ovulation.) The most familiar and widely used of these is Premarin®, a mix of what are called conjugated estrogens derived (believe it or not) from the urine of pregnant mares. (Thus the name: *Pre* for pregnant, *mar* for mare and *in* for urine.) Despite its equine origin, this preparation has held its own for years and has served as the supplement in the majority of studies which have demonstrated benefits for HRT. The typical starting dose is .625 mg., below which protection from osteoporosis is less certain. If symptom control is on the agenda, the dose may have to be increased until the offending events calm down or side effects become a problem.

Other commonly used forms of estrogen are estrone (the weaker estrogen produced by the ovaries and peripheral fat cells) which is marketed as Ogen®, and estradiol, a more potent form found in Estrace® and the Estraderm® patch. At present there is no consensus in the medical literature that one of these brands is more effective or safe than the others. Individual variations in effectiveness and side effects largely determine which of these a woman will use over the long haul.

In contrast to the estrogens, the progesterones commonly used in HRT are synthetic. Medroxyprogesterone (Provera®, Amen®, and Cycrin®) is the most widely utilized form and is effective, but may induce heavier periods than some of its relatives. Some women and their physicians are more comfortable using natural progesterone, but it must be taken by vaginal suppository, since it is not absorbed through the intestinal tract.

What about hormones for the woman who has not yet arrived at menopause?

Remember that the perimenopause may last for many months prior to the actual end of menstrual cycles, and during this time fluctuations in estrogen levels may cause not only irregular cycles, but the whole gamut of hot flashes, flushing, and sweats. Women in this situation have traditionally been in a bind, because physicians were reluctant to give any hormone supplementation to someone who was still having cycles.

Now, however, it is not uncommon to use very low dose oral contraceptives in this situation, an act that would have been considered heretical several years ago. But as long as the woman is not a smoker, and the appropriate screening has been done, this form of hormone replacement not only relieves symptoms of estrogen withdrawal but also regulates the erratic cycles.

* * *

All in all, you sound generally in favor of widespread use of hormone replacement therapy for postmenopausal women. But isn't that really tampering with the created order? As you said, menopause is a universal event, not a disease.

Indeed it is, but unfortunately it also has some consequences that can annoy or seriously impair women during a time of life that can and should be extremely productive. If we have the means to prevent some of those disturbances, and those methods appear to be safe and well-tolerated for the vast majority of women, it seems quite appropriate to utilize them.

In previous and, happily, bygone generations, some physicians believed that pain in childbirth was not only foretold in Genesis, but was also a direct expression of God's will, a punishment visited on the daughters of Eve as a reminder of her first sin. In their decidedly finite wisdom, they found it morally objectionable to offer pain relief to women in labor. Obviously, hardly anyone would accept such a notion today, nor would we find many who would object to draining swamps and killing mosquitoes (also part of the natural order) in order to prevent malaria. For that matter, acknowledging that God causes the rain to fall doesn't stop us from seeking shelter from it.

Similarly, we find it hard to believe that fractured hips and heart attacks represent an expression of God's creative design. In light of the strong evidence that hormone replacement therapies can spare millions of women needless suffering (as long as appropriate safeguards are observed), widespread use of estrogen and progesterone seems entirely appropriate.

Chapter Seven

‿◠‿◠‿

How Do I
Detect Trouble?

Most people consider a medical exam—and, in particular, one of those "stem to stern" physicals—to be about as much fun as a tax audit. But if a doctor is doing a thorough job over the long haul, time should be set aside on a regular basis for a general inspection. This should include a review of any current problems and symptoms, recommendations about any areas where there is room for improvement, and the subject of this chapter: screening for problems that might be silent but serious.

I know that check ups are a good idea. But why do doctors seem so obsessed with probing around places I'd rather have left alone?

Your lack of enthusiasm for being poked, prodded, and otherwise hassled in sensitive areas of the body is universal. But to quote the criminal who was asked why he always robbed banks, "That's where the money is." In general, the most unpleasant medical routines are those intended to ferret out cancers—specifically, those involving breast, reproductive organs, and colon. Altogether these account for about

100,000 deaths among women in the United States every year (with well over 300,000 new cases annually), not to mention untold discomfort, disruption, and expense. Many of these tumors could be caught and cured with early detection and treatment.

Assuming that I want to subject myself to these various and sundry procedures, how often should I be screened?

If you're over forty (which is likely, since not too many teenagers read books about menopause) think in terms of an annual visit for the basics (pelvic, pap smear, breast check), every two to three years for a comprehensive "State of the Union" exam, and definitely more often if advised by your physician.

Whom should I be seeing for these exams?

Traditionally, most basic screening has been done by family physicians, internists, and gynecologists, and these practitioners will continue to do so in the future, hopefully with increased vigilance as more data supports the benefits of early detection. As cost containment measures continue to affect medical care, it is possible (and in some health plans, likely) that you may be seen for routine checks by a physician's assistant or nurse practitioner. In general, these caregivers are well-trained and capable of providing excellent basic care and screening. In fact, they may spend more time, and do a better job of educating and explaining what's going on, than a physician.

Speaking of time, my doctor tears in and out of the exam room like the White Rabbit with a "very important

date"—somewhere else. Your description of a general exam with all of that detailed reviewing and recommending by the doctor sounds like some sort of fantasy. I hardly ever seem to get my questions answered, let alone any of this wise counsel. What should I do?

Unfortunately, too many doctors who are expert practitioners may also be marginal listeners and mediocre communicators. If they are also behind schedule (which is likely), you may feel that you didn't exactly "connect" during the visit. But there are a few things you can do to improve the odds of a productive visit:

1. If you have a number of things you want to talk about, let the receptionist know when you make the appointment. Every doctor hates the words "By the way... " and "While I'm here...." Often the issues you want to discuss will need much more time than a basic screening exam.

2. Bring a written "laundry list" of your questions, and let your doctor know what's on it—and what's most important to you—at the *beginning* of the visit. He or she may change the entire agenda of the visit based on that information.

3. Don't expect snappy answers to questions like, "Why am I so tired all the time?" or "What's causing my headaches?" Doctors aren't side-show psychics, and problems like these can't be addressed without a fairly detailed history and exam. If you get a quick response, it's probably not well-informed unless your doctor knows you *extremely* well.

4. If you can't get decent answers using diplomacy, subtle hints, arm-twisting, or bribery, you may need to seek care elsewhere.

**Getting back to screening. Is there really any point to it?
Sometimes I feel like the whole business is an
uncomfortable and expensive ritual.**

Good question. In fact, despite pronouncements you hear
that may sound like direct commandments from God, members
of the medical community constantly debate about the
validity and cost-effectiveness of various screening tests. But
the arguing rarely is over *whether* certain screening should be
done, but about some of the technical details: what test to use,
when to begin, how often to do it, to whom, and by whom.

**But isn't this really an exercise in futility? If you're
destined to develop a health problem (especially cancer)
at some point in life, does screening really make
any difference?**

You've touched on one of the basic philosophical issues of
screening. And while this isn't a book on public health policy,
it's worth taking a moment to look at the basic questions that
must be asked about any disease before subjecting a lot of
people to a test which screens for it.

1. Is the disease a significant cause of morbidity (a fancy word
for "being sick") or mortality (a fancy word for "being dead")?

2. Does the disease occur relatively often?

In other words, there's no point in having everyone
checked for problems that rarely cause serious harm or for
problems that are serious but highly uncommon. For example, we could propose that every young adult have a sound
wave image of the heart called an echocardiogram. It's safe, it
doesn't hurt, and we would discover a variety of abnormalities. After millions of tests were done, at a cost of billions of

dollars, we would find out, among other things, that about 10 to 15 percent of those adults have an abnormality called mitral valve prolapse, which can cause pounding sensations and chest discomfort. We would also find a very rare person with a thickening of heart muscle (called hypertrophic cardiomyopathy) that can cause sudden death.

But would all of the time, effort, and money expended to do this mass screening be worth it? For all of the prolapsed mitral valves we discovered, few (if any) would cause major trouble. The problem is common, but not exactly serious. And while it would be good to know who has the dangerous hypertrophic cardiomyopathy, literally thousands of normal people would have to be checked for every one case found, and at a huge cost.

Wait a minute—are you saying that the bottom line on screening is bucks? Isn't it worth spending any amount of money to save a life?

We always cringe when human life is devalued, as is occurring with frightening and ever increasing frequency in our once-civilized culture. God's assignment of value to a life transcends any price tag—but his resources are unlimited, and ours are not. When it comes to screening, cost *always* enters the equation (along with questions of complexity and discomfort), unless the particular test is incredibly cheap, easy, and painless. It is simply impossible to check every human being repeatedly for every possible disease that might do harm. Some lines must be drawn, and money has a way of influencing that process.

Getting back to the other questions we must ask about diseases we might screen:

3. Does the disease go through a phase where it doesn't cause symptoms or damage but can still be detected?

4. Does the disease respond better to treatment when it's detected at an early rather than an advanced stage?

In other words, it doesn't make sense to screen for a disease which can't be detected any earlier by the test than by the patient, or whose outcome is already a "done deal" no matter when you discover it. This is why, for example, many clinicians think it's a waste of time to do screening chest X-rays for lung cancer. Even though this is a common and serious disease (thus meeting the first two criteria), it's rare that you see anything on X-ray before the patient starts to have symptoms. And, once the cancer is big enough to see on X-ray, the odds of a cure are slim.

Bottom line: for a disease to be a good candidate for mass screening, it must be common, potentially serious, detectable at an early stage, and more responsive at an early stage.

Obviously, there are always individual exceptions and unusual cases, but when we talk about screening we have to think about risks, odds, statistics, and finances for tests involving *large numbers of people*. Eventually a thorny problem arises: we have to translate all of the number crunching into an individual decision: should *I* (or my mother, sister, daughter, or friend) have this or that test? Or, to put it more bluntly, is it worth the hassle, discomfort, and money to have a particular screening procedure? The final decision must always be made in light of individual circumstances and hopefully some thoughtful discussion between you and your practitioner. Therefore you should look at the information in this book—or any book that dispenses advice about health—as advisory and not dogmatic.

OK, so I want to try to head off trouble in the future. What diseases should my doctor and I be concerned about?

Thank you for reiterating a basic premise we have set forth many times already: that the years surrounding and following menopause should be great years, productive years, enjoyable years. Unfortunately, a lot of diseases that can ruin your day (or your life) tend to show up during these same years. So if you endure a minor hassle now to prevent a major hassle later, you will have taken some important steps toward that goal.

Since we've already mentioned cancer screening in this chapter, let's lead off with that unpleasant topic.

Can I ask a dumb question first? I have a vague understanding about cancer as a kind of growth that can be dangerous. But what exactly is a cancer?

To quote your tenth grade geometry teacher, there are no dumb questions. And to clear the air on cancer, you need to know another term: *neoplasm*, which literally means "new tissue." This word refers to an uncontrolled and disorderly proliferation of cells, beginning on a microscopic level but then usually noticeable in one way or another with the passage of time, at which point we refer to it as a *tumor*.

Neoplasms can cause trouble in a number of ways: by crowding out normal cells within a tissue or organ, thus interfering with its designated function; by exerting pressure on adjacent tissues or organs without actually invading them; by spreading locally and directly into nearby tissues or organs; and by spreading to distant sites (in which case the far-flung growths are called *metastases*). Neoplasms/tumors which do not invade other tissues or spread at a distance are called *benign*, while those that invade and spread are called *malignant*. The term *cancer* has been generically attached to any form of malignant growth.

Why do neoplasms form in the first place?

There is a long list of known contributors to tumor growth, but the exact cause in a given person may be difficult to determine. Genetics, environmental factors (such as excessive exposure to sunlight), contact with carcinogens (cancer-causing compounds, such as tobacco smoke), diet, viruses, the status of the immune system, and even emotions have been linked in one way or another to tumors.

What tumors should I be worried about?

To state the obvious, the most common ones. In order of frequency, the top five sites for new cancer cases in women are: breast, lung, colon, uterus (both body and cervix), and ovary.

Keep in mind that this ranking varies somewhat depending on age, and the ranking is different for causes of death. *Since the late 1980s, there are actually more deaths from lung than breast cancer, even though women with breast tumors outnumber those with lung cancer more than two to one.*

Why do such a higher percentage of women die from lung cancer?

The sad news is that less than 15 percent of people with lung cancer live more than five years once the diagnosis is made. This has to do not only with the behavior of the various lung tumors, but with the difficulty of discovering them at an early stage. Once they're big enough to show up on chest X-ray, they're usually also big enough to cause major trouble.

Furthermore, during the postwar years a lot of women bought into the exceedingly dumb idea that smoking shouldn't be the exclusive province of men. This notion was expressed for years in the "You've Come a Long Way, Baby" ads, which equated smoking with liberation from pig-brained males. The promotion of cigarette smoking is, in our humble opinion, the scum-sucking activity of bottom-feeders in the advertising food chain. It is the worst form of profiteering at the expense of untold misery and death for untold millions.

But how do you really feel? Seriously, does the evidence still link cigarette smoking and lung cancer?

Absolutely, not to mention other forms of cancer as well.

Isn't lung cancer actually starting to decline?

It is, in a sense, but only in men. Actually, what's declining in men is the *rate of increase*. (This is somewhat like the "good news" politicians offer about the national debt: it isn't growing as quickly.) Between 1950 and 1990, death rates for lung cancer in men increased fourfold. But for women, the increase was sevenfold. And while the rate of increase for men slowed in the 1980s, the rate for women increased sharply.

Since lung cancer causes the most deaths, should I have a chest X-ray every so often?

Intuitively that makes sense, but (as we mentioned earlier) routine chest X-rays on vast numbers of people rarely discover early tumors that can be cured. If you have never smoked (or stopped many years ago after a short tobacco career) and have no symptoms, a routine chest X-ray is not likely to be a profitable test. But a chest X-ray should be done if you have a prolonged, unexplained cough, shortness of breath, or a known lung disease whose progress can be followed (at least in part) by X-ray. If you are a smoker, the smartest thing you can possibly do is QUIT TODAY. And if you have a long-standing habit, your doctor may indeed suggest that you have an X-ray done every few years, despite the dismal statistics.

Other conditions may be discovered, and occasionally one of these will serve as a useful baseline for future comparisons.

Has breast cancer also been on the rise?

As we mentioned, this is the most common tumor in women, with an estimated 182,000 cases in 1993, and the leading cause of cancer death for women aged fifty to fifty-four. There was also a steady increase in the breast cancer rate (that is, number of tumors per 100,000 women) between 1940 and 1987. The sharpest rise occurred between 1982 and 1987, followed by a mild drop. These trends were partly attributable to better detection methods and more wide-spread screening in the 1980s, with more small tumors being discovered as a result. (In 1979 only 22 percent of American women reported ever having a mammogram. By 1992 that number had increased to 74 percent.)

I've heard a scary statistic that one in nine women will get breast cancer some time in her life. Is that true?

The actual statistic is that one woman in nine who is currently twenty years old and *lives to be eighty-five years old* will develop breast cancer. This is not uniform throughout life, but increases with age.

Are there any factors other than age that might put me at greater risk?

Age is clearly the most important, and 60 to 75 percent of women with breast cancer have no other known risk factors. But the following situations do increase your chances for developing this tumor:

1. A history of breast cancer in your mother or sister—or, oddly enough, a colon cancer in a parent or sibling.

2. Onset of menses before age 12.

3. Menopause after age 55. In general, a longer menstrual life increases the risk of breast cancer, but as compensation, also lowers the risk of osteoporosis.

4. No pregnancies during the reproductive years.

5. First pregnancy after age thirty. This increases the odds two- to fivefold over a woman whose first pregnancy occurs before age nineteen.

6. Premature termination of a woman's first pregnancy, whether by abortion or miscarriage. The hormonal changes of a completed pregnancy may cause increased differentiation in breast tissue (a transformation from less to more specialized cells). More differentiated tissue is less likely to undergo transformation into a cancerous growth. Abortion or miscarriage may cause the breasts to be exposed only to high estrogen levels in early pregnancy, without the hormonal advantages of the entire process.

7. A diet high in dairy and other fat may increase the risk, while Vitamin A (as little as three-quarters of a carrot every day) may reduce it.

8. Daily alcohol consumption has recently been identified as a risk factor—not the strongest, but definitely controllable. Women with other risk factors for breast cancer should consider abstaining entirely from alcohol.

What about screening for breast cancer?

Breast tumors grow very slowly, especially in their early stages, and early detection improves the odds of cure and survival. Starting in early adulthood, breast self-examination should be done at least once every month.

Why so often?

Frequent self-checks foster a familiarity with your own

breast tissue, and specifically with what is normal for you at various times of the month.

Is any particular time of the month better?

Before menopause, the breast is likely to be smoother and less lumpy during the week right after menses. But some experts suggest checking the breast every week in order to get a more complete sense of what happens during the cycle.

Speaking of bumps, my breasts are so lumpy and bumpy I can't see how I could possibly discover anything before it became the size of a walnut. What's the point of checking them?

Breasts with thicker connective tissue and lots of cysts (referred to overall as fibrocystic changes) are tougher to examine. (These changes do not lead to cancer, by the way.) But it's still wise to become an expert on your own terrain and its variations through the months and years. The object is not to develop a magical ability to know if a lump is pathological, but simply to notice if something new and different has appeared—at which point some further action can be taken with your physician. In general, breast tumors are found at earlier and more curable states among self-checkers than among their non-examining counterparts.

So how should I go about doing this?

While you don't need to make this a formal ceremony, a regular routine can take some of the apprehension out of the process. Some clinicians suggest checking once every week before you arise from bed, on whatever morning you don't have to jump out of bed at sixty miles per hour.

I don't have any mornings like that. What other bright ideas do you have?

You can try doing your monthly (or weekly) check in the shower. Some women find that they can feel with more sensitivity over a moist, soapy skin surface.

Think of each breast as divided into four sections demarcated by an imaginary horizontal and vertical line, with the upper outer section including a "tail" that extends toward the armpit. Gently feel the four quadrants of each breast with the opposite hand, using the flat part of the middle fingers and not just the tips.

How about letting my husband do this for me?

He may have difficulty keeping his mind on the purpose of the exam! But if he's interested and careful, he could easily become an adept examiner. Nevertheless, it would be wise for you to do your own checks as well.

The whole idea of self-checking makes me nervous. I know I'm going to find lumps and bumps that will scare me, and then I'll be running to the doctor every other week.

This is why you need to become acquainted with your personal geography. Remember that you can wait a week or two and then check again. Some bumps ebb and flow during the cycle, so what feels worrisome today may soon be gone. You can also try a few self-checks before your next exam, and then compare notes with your doctor.

The regular exam by your primary care provider should definitely be a yearly routine for anyone over forty, and certainly an accompaniment to a pelvic exam/pap smear (see below) at any age. A breast exam by an experienced practitioner may uncover a suspicious lump that you have missed, and even one that a mammogram cannot detect.

Speaking of mammograms, what's the point of subjecting the breasts to a lot of radiation over a period of years? Can that in itself cause cancer?

Mammography techniques have improved significantly over the past several years, increasing detail and decreasing radiation exposure to a negligible level. The main issues now have to do with how often and when, not any risk of the procedure itself.

I've read about some controversies regarding mammograms. Can't you doctors agree on anything?

Like we said earlier, recommendations and guidelines aren't set in concrete, and reputable organizations do not always come to the same conclusions. Mammography (along with ultrasound imaging, when appropriate) can help determine whether a mass that someone has felt is likely to be benign or not. But the controversy is *screening* mammography, whose purpose is to detect tumors that are too small to be felt even by the most brilliant clinician. Remember that breast tumors, in their earliest phases, grow very slowly; it may take as long as five years before a tumor is big enough to feel. But the window of time during which a growth is big enough to be seen on a mammogram but still too small to be felt may last anywhere from *eighteen months to four years.* And during that time the cancer has had plenty of time to send its grubby little malignant cells to other parts of the body. Finding a cancer at an early stage, before it has had time to spread, can be life-saving.

Sounds like a great idea to me. So what's the problem?

Annual mammograms are definitely a great idea for women fifty and over. Nearly every major medical organization, including the American Cancer Society and the National Cancer Institute, endorse annual mammograms between ages fifty and seventy-five, with estimates that doing so could cut death rates from breast cancer by 30 percent. For women between the ages of forty and forty-nine, mammograms every one to two years have been traditionally recommended. But there is now dissent in the ranks.

The problem is that suspicious areas on mammograms usually lead to local biopsies, many of which turn out to be negative for cancer. In such cases the mammogram result is called a "false positive." The end result is obviously good news for the patient, but a fair amount of effort, time, expense, and worry has also taken place. This is particularly an issue for women younger than fifty, for whom breast tissue tends to be thicker and more difficult to interpret on a mammogram. And in these days of medical cost-containment, more than a few bean-counters have been reviewing how many of these false alarm scenarios take place—and how much they cost— for every real tumor that is found. It turns out that, from this perspective, mammograms are more cost-effective in women fifty and over than in their younger counterparts, except for those with a family history of breast cancer.

In addition, some research—especially a large study from Canada called the Canadian National Breast Screening Study, and a major analysis of eight studies called the "Fletcher Report"—has suggested that screening women in their forties doesn't improve overall death rates. But other studies have shown improved survival, and some stinging criticisms have been fired at the design and execution of the Canadian study. The American Cancer Society, sticking to its traditional guns, points out that one in six cases of breast cancer occurs in women in their forties and that dropping recommendations for screening younger women will inevitably lead to lack of insurance coverage for them.

This all sounds totally confusing, like a bunch of theologians arguing over some interpretation of Scripture. How am I supposed to make an intelligent decision in the face of this controversy?

First of all, don't forget the basics: monthly self-checking, annual breast exams, and annual mammograms after age fifty. If you are in your forties, a mammogram every two years should definitely be considered, especially if you have one or more risk factors. If there is a history of breast cancer in your mother or one or more sisters, there should be no question about early screening because your risk is advanced about ten years compared to your peer age group. (That is, if you are forty, you carry the risk of a fifty-year-old.)

It seems smarter at this time to err on the side of more rather than less frequent mammography, whether or not insurance foots the bill. While statistics and mass population trends are important, no statistician will appear at your bedside to offer condolences if a cancer is diagnosed too late.

What if a suspicious lump is revealed by manual examination or a mammogram?

The entire range of diagnostic and therapeutic strategies is way beyond the scope and intent of this book. But, as a bottom line, don't back away from finding out what is going on. In some cases it may be appropriate to watch a lump for one cycle to see if it changes drastically or disappears. But overall, knowing is better than not knowing, and earlier is better than later.

What action your primary care doctor or a general surgeon might choose will depend on a host of factors. You should not expect instant answers because solving the problem will take time. And you should not accept any medical intervention without a chance to hear and consider all the options. The old horror stories about women feeling a lump in the morning and having a mastectomy that afternoon are a thing of the not-so-dearly departed past. There are no emergencies in diagnosing and treating breast tumors and no need to make snap decisions. If you feel you need time to think, take it. If you want another opinion, get it. But don't fall into the trap of "doctor shopping" to find someone who will offer what seems to be the least unsettling recommendations.

Moving right along, what other screening delights should I look forward to during a complete exam?

By now, most women are accustomed to having pelvic exams and pap smears done on a routine basis, even though they loathe them.

You got that right. Why do we put up with these yearly intrusions, anyway?

No one says you have to, although few doctors will prescribe oral contraceptives or hormone replacement without checking the anatomy first. As with the other tests and exams, the primary purpose is to look for all sorts of abnormalities, and especially to detect cancers at earlier and more treatable stages.

In case you're one of the few women who hasn't had the exciting experience of a pelvic exam, this procedure normally involves three phases. First, one must assume an uncomfortable position with feet in ice cold stirrups, knees bent, legs far enough apart to strain the hip joints, and fanny hanging in the breeze (though with a sheet over your pelvis and knees, like a tent) at the end of an exam table.

Second, a plastic or metal duckbill-shaped device called a speculum is inserted into the vagina. (If made of metal, the speculum usually seems to come directly from the refrigerator.) This allows inspection of the outer genital area, vagina, and cervix, which is the opening of the uterus into the vagina. The cells in this area undergo rapid turnover, and they may begin to show a number of abnormalities before an actual cancer is present. It is relatively easy during a pelvic check to scrape some cells from the cervix with a wooden spatula and a small brush, smear them on a slide and send them to a lab for review. Dr. G.N. Papanicolaou introduced this concept of screening during the early 1940s, and his name has become synonymous with the procedure women love to hate. (At the same time, cells are also scraped from the vagina, even though it is an uncommon site for cancer.)

What happens if these slides look abnormal?

The most common abnormalities are actually not impending cancerous changes but less ominous cell changes caused by inflammation or hormonal factors. Usually these are simply rechecked in a few months. If abnormalities persist or worsen, a physician (almost always a gynecologist) will examine the cervix more carefully using some special stains and fancy optical equipment called a colposcope. Often small samples of tissue (biopsies) are taken and sent to the lab. Treatment will depend upon the findings, and often with these techniques very early cancers are discovered and eliminated.

How often should I put up with a pap smear?

The answer depends on who you ask. Most physicians recommend that a pelvic and pap smear be done annually on women starting at age twenty, or sooner if they are sexually active.

Why is that? I thought that cancer in this area was a problem for older women.

Not so. There is now ample evidence linking cancer of the cervix, and its preliminary changes, to certain forms of a sexually-transmitted virus known as HPV, the human papilloma virus. Women who begin having sex in their early teens and those with multiple partners are at much higher risk of developing ominous cellular changes, and even full-blown cancer, at an early age. Those who wait until marriage to have sex, and remain in a mutually exclusive relationship, have much less to worry about, although the regular check is still wise.

I've heard about some recommendations that the pap could be done only every three years. Why do it more often?

A number of national organizations, including the American Cancer Society, have suggested that after three consecutive normal paps, the smear can be done less often (meaning every two to three years) "at the discretion of the physician." Most primary care doctors and gynecologists balk at this advice—not because they need to see more patients, but because the pap smear can change drastically in a year's time. Also, the pap is simple, harmless, and relatively inexpensive, and a number of other worthwhile health screening activities usually take place at the same time.

Such as...?

Such as breast checks, blood pressure screening, and discussions of smoking, exercise, lifestyle, and so forth, depending on the time allotted for the visit.

What if I've had a hysterectomy?

A pap smear should still be taken from the upper end of the vagina every three years, and the pelvic and other screening exams are worthwhile annually.

You said there were three phases of the pelvic check. What's the third?

The examiner inserts two fingers of one hand into the vagina (wearing a latex glove, of course) and presses externally over the pelvis with the other. Aside from generating a feeling of imminent need to pass urine, this allows a quick check of the size and shape of the body of the uterus and the ovaries on either side of it. Any enlargement, tenderness, or other abnormal findings should be chased down with other studies. For example, if either ovary feels enlarged, a pelvic ultrasound or computerized tomography (or CT, a cross-sectional X-ray procedure) may be an appropriate next step. The rectal exam is commonly, but not always, the grand finale of the exam.

Is there any way to screen for early cancers in the ovaries?

Unfortunately, pelvic examination is not terribly sensitive, and an ovary must be fairly large to be readily felt. (If a woman is obese, even a huge growth may be difficult to feel.) And, unlike the cervix and breast, the available screening methods for the ovary are either marginally reliable or expensive and complicated.

A blood test known as CA-125, if elevated, may indicate an ovarian cancer is present, but several other tumors and unrelated conditions (for example, liver disease) may elevate it also. This test is most useful in a supporting role, not as the main event in screening. On the other hand, sound wave imaging using a vaginal probe can accurately evaluate the size and shape of ovaries and their blood flow patterns. Such tests are safe and (believe it or not) well-accepted by women, but they are expensive—in the $700 range for the full sound wave exam. Since it is impractical to screen every woman with these studies, most physicians agree that women with a *positive family history for cancer of the ovary* should definitely have the CA-125 and vaginal ultrasound studies, if possible at an age younger than that at which the relative developed the disease.

Is there a similar sort of problem screening the colon?

To some extent, yes. You won't typically have symptoms from a colon cancer, and a doctor will rarely feel it on routine exam, unless it is huge. Ideally, it would be extremely helpful if every adult could have a full colon exam using a fiberoptic scope (known as colonoscopy) at least once during mid-life, if not more often. But there aren't enough gastroenterologists nor enough bucks (at several hundred dollars per procedure) available to do this on a mass scale.

So what's the alternative?

The majority of colon tumors are found in the last several inches of the colon (called the sigmoid, because its shape resembles the letter "s"). An inspection of this area on a regular basis takes only a few minutes.

Wait a minute... This sounds pretty unpleasant.

Don't panic. The instrument that does the looking is called a sigmoidoscope, a flexible thin fiberoptic tube that is guided by a physician on a journey lasting only a few minutes. The sensation for most is mildly unpleasant, somewhat like a bowel movement punctuated by a brief cramp or two. A few people, if they are prone to spasm in the colon, may feel more significant cramping. This experience does not require sedation or any preparation other than a couple of Fleet's enemas just before the procedure.

And how often should this wonderful event take place?

Physicians usually recommend having a sigmoidoscopy for two consecutive years starting at age fifty, and then every three to five years thereafter.

Why the two consecutive years first?

Theoretically, if the examiner doesn't spot a small growth the first time around, he or she probably will one year later. If nothing interesting is seen twice in a row, the odds are slim that anything has been missed, and the less frequent schedule can be continued.

What exactly is the doctor looking for?

Primarily for small growths called polyps, which have a tendency to turn into tumors as the years pass. If one of these little wads of tissue is found, it will be removed (usually by snaring and snipping with a thin wire), then sent to the pathologist. If the polyp is too large to be treated through the scope, or a more ominous mass is found, a biopsy can be taken—but nearly always some sort of surgical follow-up is needed.

What about the rest of the colon?

Some people need to have the entire colon inspected, using a longer instrument called a colonoscope. As might be expected, this procedure is a bigger deal than a sigmoidoscopy, requiring a more detailed consultation by a gastroenterologist beforehand and intravenous sedation during the procedure. Since the examinee is conked out for most of the proceedings, the biggest complaint is always about the process of flushing out the entire colon ahead of time. This bowel prep involves downing four liters (about a gallon) of a special solution the day before, and then spending a fair amount of time in the bathroom.

Sounds great. How do I qualify for this experience?

The people who should have a colonoscopy are those who have one or more of the following warning signs: a parent or sibling with colon cancer (this is yet another disease with links in the family tree); family members with multiple polyps; an ongoing problem with ulcerative colitis (*not* the garden variety irritable colon, which carries no cancer risk); polyps found on a sigmoidoscopy (if there's one below, there may be more farther up); and, most commonly, occult blood in the stool.

I don't think I want to know, but how does one check for occult blood (whatever that is) in the stool?

Occult literally means *hidden*. Most people will (and should) quickly seek medical help if they see blood in the toilet bowl. But cancers and polyps frequently ooze small amounts of blood which are detectable chemically but not visually. By age fifty (and probably sooner), every year your doctor should hand you a little "stool kit," which allows you the pleasant task of poking at three different bowel movements with little sticks and transferring small samples onto a special card. When three of these are completed, a special solution is dripped onto the other side of the card. A color change indicates (usually) that blood is lurking in the stool.

(Eating a lot of rare meat, or consuming aspirin prior to the test, may produce a false positive.)

Yuck! This sounds disgusting. Do I really have to do this?

Like everything else we've discussed, it's a free country. This is without a doubt the screening that everyone most dislikes, that gets lost in the shuffle, that is conveniently ignored and forgotten. But the 75,000 women every year who discover they have a colon tumor—and the families of the nearly 30,000 who will die—won't be able to ignore this problem. This is one cancer where an early interception can make a serious difference.

This is getting a little morbid. Aren't you spending an awful lot of time talking about cancer?

Only because the screening tests for these common tumors are the most unpleasant and thus the most easily avoided. Now that we've beaten them into the ground, we should move on to some other important matters which are a little easier to screen.

Such as..?

Cardiovascular risk factors. We've already talked about the serious problem of coronary artery disease and the importance of being "heart smart," which includes knowing where you stand. As we spelled out in Chapter Three, you should know your *total and HDL cholesterol levels* like your phone number. You should have your *blood pressure* checked regularly—an easy process every time you have a checkup, donate blood, or even have your teeth cleaned. You will probably know without asking whether your *weight* is higher than desirable, but a discussion with your physician may be appropriate to set a reasonable target and a realistic time frame to get there with an appropriate approach.

What about an electrocardiogram (ECG) or a treadmill test?

These are not automatic screening items on every physical. Determining if and when to do either will depend on several factors. If you are the proud owner of a number of risk factors for coronary artery disease (run back to Chapter Three, if you don't remember), a more thorough assessment of your heart's status and performance may be in order.

Does having a normal ECG mean that my heart is OK?

Unfortunately not. The resting electrocardiogram is an electrical portrait of your heart, which may (among many other things) show if you have killed some heart muscle in the past, or if the heart has had to build up its muscle to compensate for prolonged high blood pressure. But you can have a completely normal ECG with coronary arteries that are ready to close off at any moment.

That's reassuring. What's the point of having one?

At some point, if nothing else, it's nice to have a baseline for future comparison. Many times a slightly abnormal ECG during a period of chest discomfort can be difficult to interpret, and a prior tracing, done when things were calm, can be extremely useful. Unfortunately, not many insurance companies will pay for such information, even if you have a stack of risk factors.

What about the treadmill? What does that show?

A treadmill takes a look at the heart's performance during

exercise. ECG electrodes are placed on the arms, legs and chest (they don't hurt, by the way), and then you begin to walk—first at a very slow pace, then at a faster rate, then with the treadmill tilted slightly uphill. The heart rate and blood pressure are closely monitored, and the tracing is observed for changes which suggest that the heart isn't happy with the blood it's receiving. Pain in the chest may also send that message.

A treadmill can be useful in sorting out the cause of chest pain, especially if the pattern is unusual or confusing. It also should be done if you are over forty and considering a significant upgrade in your exercise. Most people don't need this if they simply plan to begin a conservative walking program. But if you plan to begin some form of vigorous (hopefully supervised) conditioning, a treadmill test can be a wise investment.

Is there any danger involved in a treadmill? I don't want to drop dead while I'm trying to improve my health!

The actual physical risk of a properly supervised treadmill is extremely low. (This is assuming, of course, that you are dealing with a well-trained technician and the supervising physician is present or in the facility; that standard protocols are being followed; and that the test is terminated if certain warning signs are noted.) The most common problem with treadmill tests is with equivocal results. A fair number of abnormal results in people with no symptoms turn out to be "false positives." That is, further testing indicates that nothing apparently is wrong. Unfortunately, a fair amount of expense and anxiety may be generated before the question is settled.

Let's get back to something a little less complicated. How about any other lab tests?

A screening lab panel is often done as part of a general

exam. Whether this should be done every few years or every few months will have to be individualized. But some useful information to check every three years or so includes:

1. Glucose (or "blood sugar"). Diabetes sneaks up on many people without any symptoms at all, especially in those who are overweight. This is the so-called "adult onset" diabetes, which accounts for 80 percent of all cases. It does not require insulin to survive, but can produce a number of horrendous long-term complications. These may include accelerated coronary disease, blindness, kidney failure, loss of circulation leading to amputation of feet or legs, and disorders of the nervous system and digestion. It is extremely important to bring the glucose down toward the normal range as soon as possible. Usually this is accomplished with diet and exercise, but medications may be necessary as well.

2. Blood count. A low red cell count (anemia) not only can cause fatigue, but may indicate iron deficiency and trigger a search for blood loss (especially from the colon). Many cases of colon cancer have been discovered because of an unexpected anemia found on a routine blood count.

3. Iron level. Iron deficiency frequently precedes anemia and likewise may signal the need to search for blood loss. (In a woman with extremely heavy periods, the answer may be obvious, and the iron deficiency then serves to indicate how serious the problem has become.)

4. Urinalysis. Occasionally a routine urinalysis will reveal an unsuspected bladder infection, contain glucose that signals the presence of diabetes, or contain protein that reflects any number of problems in the kidney. In addition, the presence of an abnormal number of red blood cells in the urine should *always* be evaluated fully, unless it can be proven that the specimen was contaminated by blood from a menstrual flow. This could be the first and only sign, until things are much more advanced, of a tumor in the bladder or kidney.

5. Thyroid hormone levels. Usually there will be a variety of symptoms if the thyroid is over or underactive, although these may not be very specific. When menstrual periods change unexpectedly, a check of thyroid hormone isn't a bad idea (along with more direct assessments of the reproductive system).

This screening business seems like quite a project. Who's going to pay for all of these wonderful tests?

A very good, and sticky, question. Some enlightened insurance plans actually allow coverage for these procedures, at a reasonable frequency. But others don't contribute a nickel, or they make you jump through all sorts of hoops to get what you want or need.

If you find that you are footing the entire bill yourself, don't forget that you don't necessarily need to do everything at once. A little planning with your physician can usually parcel your particular "laundry list" into workable installments over the course of a year, covering the most important areas first. Some of these tests can be done for a nominal fee at a local health fair. And radiology facilities will often run "specials" on mammography at certain times of the year.

One other thought: you wouldn't hesitate to shop for the best price for a television or some new furniture. Likewise, if you are not constrained by your insurance policy to use certain providers, don't be afraid to inquire around town for the current costs of some of the procedures we have discussed. You may be surprised at how much the price of a treadmill or a sigmoidoscopy may vary within a community.

Any parting shots?

Nice pun. Don't forget to update your tetanus shot every ten years, or after five years if you suffer a dirty wound. Also, consider a flu shot every fall if you are over fifty-five, or if you have some ongoing health problem such as chronic lung disease or diabetes. A red hot case of influenza is a real drag (fever, cough, terrible aches, feeling as though you've been hit by a truck) and may generate some important complications if your health isn't great to begin with.

Well, I must say you've given me a lot to think about. I may need some of those anti-depressants you discussed earlier—some of this is pretty depressing.

Sorry, it's just part of the job. But stick around; the good stuff comes next.

What "good stuff" might that be? More warning labels to paste on various parts of my body?

Nope. The *really* good stuff. The stuff you've been waiting for.... unless you already skipped ahead, of course. The next chapter is on—you guessed it—sex.

It's about time. Maybe I should stick around a little longer....

Chapter Eight

ᥣᥬᥓᥬᥱ

Is There (Sex) Life
After 50?

Can we talk?
About what?
About sex.
[*Silence*]

And that, dear friends, illustrates a major problem with sex. Most of us cannot comfortably discuss sex—and especially our *own* sexuality—at *any* age, much less around midlife and beyond when (mythically) we're not supposed to be interested in sex any more. Well, here comes a news flash (and not just a hot flash): an active, satisfying sex life long after age fifty is not only worth talking about, but is both possible and very natural.

Note to the reader:

For the majority of this book, you have been reading what amounts to a dialogue between an anonymous woman and Paul and Teri. But because one woman cannot possibly represent the vast diversity of sexual issues and experiences, we will open up this discussion to more anonymous women. Hopefully, one of them will represent you.

Some of you are thinking, "Oh good ... 'cause it sure ain't so active right now." And others are thinking, "Oh mercy....and I was looking forward to a well-earned rest from all that!" Well, you can relax, because the bottom-line message of this chapter is that sexuality in later years can be alive and well *at what - ever level* you and your spouse choose to experience it. The Duke Center for the Study of Aging and Human Development began a study in 1954 which discovered that sexual interest *and* capacity persisted into the *ninth decade* of individuals who have reasonably good physical and psychological health.

What are you talking about? My parents are well into their seventies, and I can't conceive of them "carrying on" at this point in their lives!

Adult children are often uncomfortable with the thought that their aging parents might still be sexually active. But the fact is that interest, frequency, and enjoyment of sexual expression all continue for many people well into their later years, especially if satisfying sex has been a reality during their younger years. One 1988 study detailed the sexual activity of 80 to 102-year-olds! (Of course, toward the century mark, there's a lot more cuddling and fewer orgasms.)

Does this mean that every person over age sixty is enjoying a secret life of wild sexual abandon?

Well, not exactly. According to the Stanford Menopause Study, which was launched in 1979, 48 percent of post-menopausal women reported a *decline* in sexual interest, while 29 percent reported no change, and 23 percent reported an increase.

Now I'm confused. Are you saying that sexual desire increases or decreases during and after menopause?

It all depends on the individual. Human sexuality is extremely complicated, involving not only biological factors, but psychological, emotional, and even spiritual factors as well. There are, for example, many reasons why some women report lower levels of sexual desire during and after menopause:

1. **Disruptive symptoms of falling estrogen levels** such as tiredness from night sweats and interrupted sleep, vaginal dryness, and so on. (These would have slowed down even Marilyn Monroe.)
2. **Fear of a mid-life pregnancy** just as the last child has been successfully ushered (at least temporarily) out the door.
3. **Negative cultural feedback about sexuality in older women.** The stereotype says they're not interested any more, leading a postmenopausal woman to the unfortunate expectation that libido is *supposed* to wane.
4. **Loss of partner.** Contrary to what the media would have us believe, emotionally healthy people experience desire most readily in the context of a committed, secure relationship. For many widows, sexual desire departs with the loss of the one whose bed she has shared for so many years.
5. **Loss of partner's health** through chronic illness or disability.
6. **Unresolved lifelong conflicts with one's partner.** Women of any age generally resent having intercourse with a man with whom they have a bad relationship.
7. **Sexual hang-ups from childhood.** Early taboos and negative messages about sex lead to a pattern of enduring rather than enjoying sex and a desire to phase out intercourse as soon as conveniently possible.

8. **Emotional scarring from hysterectomy or mastectomy,** which can cause feelings of being "neutered" and sexually unattractive.

9. **Attitudes connecting body image with libido.** The belief that one must have a twenty-one-year-old body in order to be sexy can hamper healthy sex.

Bingo—Number One on your list is my big problem! I used to have plenty of sexual desire, but lately it just plain hurts most of the time during intercourse, and my enthusiasm is fast waning! What's going on?

One of the most common reasons is atrophic vaginitis—some textbooks call it "senile" vaginitis. (Doesn't that sound sexy?) No wonder we have an image of middle-aged women being sexless. Somehow, having one's vagina labeled as "senile" before the other faculties qualify for this term isn't exactly encouraging.

During young adulthood, the vaginal walls serve as a kind of cushion during intercourse, protecting the bladder and urethra. But as levels of estrogen slowly drop before and after menopause, the vaginal walls become much thinner. Adding insult to injury, vaginal lubrication becomes much less abundant. A relatively speedy fifteen to thirty seconds to become moist when stimulated becomes a much more leisurely five to ten minutes after menopause. This lack of moisture, and a more acidic environment, results in vulnerability to local infections by yeast and bacteria.

All this can add up to vaginal dryness, itching, and sometimes even bleeding during intercourse. Like any other uncomfortable event, painful sex sends a blunt message to the brain: "Please do not repeat this experience!" After a few more rounds of such misery, the sex drive can be knocked out of the best of us. As one woman put it, "The week after my period, I was always eager to make love with my husband. But now sex is *flat*, and part of the problem is knowing that it's going to hurt!"

In addition, postmenopausal estrogen loss can cause the uterus to shrink somewhat, and contractions of uterine muscle that used to be smooth and pleasurable during orgasm can now become spasmodic and painful.

By the way, even though these common changes can lead to painful intercourse, this symptom should never be ignored. Other possible causes such as endometriosis (the abnormal presence of displaced uterine tissue in the pelvis), infection, or even tumor are important problems which require medical attention.

**This all sounds pretty revolting! Isn't there anything
I can do to combat "vaginal atrophy" and other irritants?**

Absolutely. First, resurrect the Kegel exercises you should have been taught during pregnancy (assuming, of course, that you had this experience) and do them with a vengeance while you read the rest of this chapter. These strengthen the "hammock" of muscles (*pubococcygeals*) which support the pelvic organs and vaginal tissue. They also maintain strength and responsiveness of the vaginal wall.

**Sorry, the memory escapes me.
How do I do Kegel exercises?**

It's quite simple: the next time you urinate, try to stop the flow of urine before the stream ends. Hold it for a count of three, and then let go. The tightening of the muscles you just employed constitute a Kegel exercise. To strengthen the pelvic floor, you need to repeat this several dozen times a day.

I don't visit the bathroom that often!

Let's hope not. But you don't have to be passing urine to tighten the muscles. Try doing 10 Kegel contractions every time you come to a red light or at every commercial break you hear on TV or radio. If you persist in doing these, you will not only improve sexual pleasure and responsiveness, but also help prevent the sagging of the pelvic structures that leads to stress incontinence.

Second, as we already mentioned in Chapter Six, estrogen replacement restores the thickness and mucus production of the vaginal walls. Oral, patch, and vaginal cream forms are all effective for this purpose. The Yale University Study on Sexual Problems During Menopause showed that 90 percent of women reported an increase in their sexual desire after three to six months of hormonal treatment.

Third, don't forget the old standbys: the over-the-counter lubricants such as K-Y Jelly®, which have proven to be quite effective for decades. (Make sure you don't use a petroleum-based product, by the way.)

The fourth solution is one your husband will probably endorse, but you might want to finish reading this section before you call him in. Several reports, including a 1991 study at the Robert Wood Johnson Medical School in New Jersey, show a direct correlation between continued sexual activity and both desire *and* enjoyment of sexual intercourse. In addition, pelvic exams showed that those who had consistently maintained sexual activity over the years showed fewer signs of vaginal atrophy.

Other studies have shown that consistent sexual activity throughout menopause (a minimum of three times a month, so we're not talking about spending your life in a negligee) seems to help preserve functioning and may even stimulate estrogen production. (Of course, there's always the possibility that all this was cooked up by some sexually frustrated researcher who was the husband of a menopausal woman....)

Lastly, we need to raise a simple but important question: if it takes longer to get lubricated, SO WHAT? This can induce your husband to put a little romance into the sexual relationship—it's called foreplay, in case you've forgotten. Teach him what you need, and maybe you'll find out what a delightfully fast learner he can be!

I can relate to the second item on your list of reasons why women no longer feel a strong sex drive. I'm forty-nine and my periods have been erratic for several years. In fact, they have all but stopped. But I just can't relax during lovemaking, knowing there's always a possibility that a little bundle of joy might arrive on my fiftieth birthday. When am I truly out of the woods regarding pregnancy?

Because you never say "never" in medicine, no one can tell you, with 100 percent assurance, that you are no longer capable of having a baby—unless you've had a hysterectomy! Having said that, a six month lapse in menstrual cycles is a pretty safe bet, and a one year hiatus even more so, especially if a confirmatory FSH blood test is elevated into the postmenopausal range (see Chapter Two).

That's not exactly helpful if I am having a period now and again. What about birth control at this time in my life?

This is a topic best suited for a conversation with your physician, because specific details about your anatomy and physiology enter the equation. But in a nutshell, you can still use most of the methods that have been devised to prevent egg and sperm from getting acquainted. These include the barrier methods (foam, condoms, diaphragm) and even (believe it or not) the birth control pill.

A decade ago it would have been heretical to prescribe oral contraceptives for women over forty. But now certain low-dose brands are used all the way into menopause without difficulty. This requires, of course, appropriate physical screening (including pap smear, breast check, and possibly mammography). This method is absolutely not for smokers, and not advisable for women with high blood pressure or a history of clot formation in the past.

Also, your husband might be a candidate (if he doesn't chicken out) for a vasectomy, especially if none of the current methods are possible or acceptable to you.

Speaking of my husband, he had a heart attack last year, and now whenever we make love I'm scared that something may happen. How am I supposed to relax and enjoy sex when I'm worried that it might kill him?

Men between the ages of forty-five and sixty have coronary artery disease at nearly three times the rate of women in the same age group. Thus it's not unusual for a woman in her middle years to have gone through the agonizing experience of watching her husband suffer, and hopefully recover from, a heart attack. The scare generated by the thought of losing your mate is terrifying, and most couples reduce or stop all sexual activity after a heart attack for fear of precipitating another one.

Lovemaking lasts, on the average, ten to fifteen minutes. The heart rate increases to 90 to 160 beats per minute, which is the range for moderate physical exercise. While your husband will want to abide strictly by his doctor's recommendations, the ability to climb a flight of stairs without distress usually means it is safe to resume normal sexual activity. (One way for the man to conserve energy during intercourse, by the way, is for the woman to be on top.)

As much as we may dislike it, our advancing years often signal the coming of medical problems which can interfere with activities we used to enjoy. But so *much* can be done, especially during the decades prior to menopause, to reduce the risk for the most common chronic illnesses. Since most of you skipped Chapter Three (because it contains boring topics like exercise and nutrition) to get to the good stuff, we want to encourage you to go back and devour that material! Sexual activity can certainly be adapted to accommodate various illnesses of later years, but a little preventive work can go a long way toward making this unnecessary.

You mentioned feeling "neutered" by a hysterectomy, and I can really relate to that. I had a partial hysterectomy six months ago, and I've been depressed ever since. Will I ever feel (sexually) normal again?

Depending on whose research you examine, it is estimated that 40 to 50 percent of all women will undergo a so-called partial (uterus only) or complete (uterus *and* ovaries) hysterectomy by age sixty-five. Teri had to have a partial hysterectomy at age twenty-eight because of complications of her second pregnancy, and she woke up in the recovery room with a very deep and completely unanticipated depression. After years of talking to women of all ages, she now realizes that her reaction was normal, and not just a result of her young age. Whether twenty-five or sixty-five, a woman who loses her reproductive organs initially experiences a tremendous sense of loss, even when she is older and knows rationally that her childbearing days have long been over. At any age, we pass through a time of asking "Am I still a woman?" and wondering if our husbands still find us attractive.

We absolutely recommend that a woman be prepared emotionally *prior* to a hysterectomy, if possible. She needs to know that the "neutered" feeling eventually passes, after appropriately grieving for the loss of her fertility (assuming that her cycles were still continuing at the time of the surgery). Most women, once fully recovered, find that freedom from concern about pregnancy can help add a wonderful sense of relaxation to the whole sexual encounter.

Two specific post-hysterectomy sexual issues should be mentioned. First, be aware that the vagina has probably been slightly shortened during the surgery, and intercourse might be a little painful at first. Sexual intercourse should NOT be attempted until the suture line in the back of the vagina has had plenty of time to heal (at least six to eight weeks after surgery). When lovemaking does resume, it needs to be extremely slow and gentle the first several times while the vagina is stretching out to once again accommodate your husband's penis.

Second, some women depend on uterine contractions to achieve orgasm. If you are in this category, and are willing to creatively experiment with more clitoral stimulation, you *will* find a new route to the same destination.

Since you brought it up, I have never had the nerve to talk to anyone about orgasms, and I'm embarrassed to say how little I know at my age! Can we take a brief detour to educate me a little bit about what to expect in this department as I get older?

It never ceases to amaze us that, in our age of sexually-explicit discussions in women's magazines, talk shows, and even public schools, so few women are sure if or when they've ever had an orgasm, or how to repeat the experience.

For the record, the female orgasm is the phase of a sexual encounter during which a peak of intense pleasure occurs. It is a specific physical event (you *know* if you've had one) accompanied by involuntary contractions of the uterus and the muscles surrounding the vagina. Unlike the male sexual climax, which is directly correlated with ejaculation of semen and intensely focused in the genital area, a woman's orgasm encompasses the entire body. And while a man requires a period of time to "re-charge" before he can experience a full orgasm again, a woman can be brought to this point repeatedly during one sexual encounter. While an orgasmic event is not necessary for a woman to enjoy sex, the feeling of satisfaction and subsequent relaxation is unlike any other sensation a woman experiences.

For the past three decades, a debate has raged about whether women experience one or two kinds of orgasms—clitoral or vaginal. (Definitions again: the clitoris is the highly sensitive organ located just above the urethra, the tube through which urine is passed. It correlates anatomically with the male penis, including the ability to become erect, and is designed solely for sexual pleasure.) Based on Teri's counseling experience, the debate appears to go on mainly among researchers in white lab coats, because the vast majority of women (those who will talk about it) say without question that their orgasm is chiefly a function of clitoral stimulation, either during intercourse or by manual stimulation. And the clitoris *remains* the primary organ of sexual excitement whether you are 22 or 102 years old, which is why a woman is theoretically capable of having an orgasm at 102. When you have an orgasm, you experience a series of contractions which move down the vagina. The *duration* of an orgasm is going to drop measurably between the ages of fifty and seventy because the *number* of uterine and vaginal contractions during an orgasm is reduced. Uterine contractions drop from three to five down to one or two per orgasm; vaginal contractions may decrease to four or five per orgasm, down from eight to twelve earlier in life.) But the good news is that a woman at *any* age retains the ability to experience one or more multiple orgasms within one lovemaking session, so cheer up!

Let's get back to a less pleasant topic: the effect of surgeries on sex. One of my big worries about being checked for breast cancer is that I might find out I need

a mastectomy. And I feel like our sex life would come to a screeching halt if that occurred.

Mastectomy is an even deeper source of psychological pain in terms of a woman's perception of her attractiveness. Whereas hysterectomy leaves no outward scars, the loss of one or two breasts—in a society which puts so much value on cleavage—can be utterly devastating to a woman's sexual confidence. But you need to keep the big picture in perspective. First of all, do not let your fears about a possible cancer diagnosis prevent you from getting routine checks! A long delay of the "ignorance is bliss" variety could actually *create* the need for a more involved surgical procedure if one became necessary.

Breast cancer is not uniformly treated by surgically removing the breast. If you are told that surgery is advisable, you must also be given full information about alternatives and their outcomes. (In fact, some states *require by law* that this information be given to a woman with breast cancer.) If, for whatever reason, you are having problems getting the information you need, you can call the National Cancer Institute cancer hot line at 1-800-4-CANCER. And you might want to think about getting another opinion.

If you are ever diagnosed as having a breast cancer, and the best chances of survival involve a mastectomy, breast reconstruction should be thoroughly discussed at the same time. If you are a candidate for reconstruction, *don't let your age be a factor weighing against your decision.*

Also, because mastectomies are not rare, support groups are available in most communities. It would be wise to contact one of them *prior* to the procedure, and hopefully both you and your husband could be better prepared as a result. (For information about local support, contact Reach for Recovery at 1-800-ACS-2345 or The Susan G. Komen Breast Cancer Foundation at 1-800-IM-AWARE.)

Needless to say, mastectomy does not signal the end of sexuality. Some women use a prosthesis (padded bra) during lovemaking initially because they are self-conscious. But as an understanding husband tenderly explores the scarred area and reassures his wife that the removal of a breast has not affected his desire for her, the prognosis for the resumption of a healthy sex life can be very good.

I haven't experienced anything so dramatic—I just haven't felt very sexy in the past few years. My breasts sag, I've put on weight, and my neck is wrinkled. There's no way my husband could be turned on by this current package. The poor guy must really be desperate to be so persistent in his amorous efforts!

Yes, feeling attractive and sexy is an important part of enjoying sex, and in this youth-obsessed culture, aging women can certainly feel left out. But why do you assume that your partner no longer finds you sexually attractive just because you're no longer young? Don't make the mistake of measuring yourself by the tiresome standards of the young, whose focus all too often can be on appearance and performance. The sexual activity of your middle years is slower and much more delicious—measured in terms of *quality* rather than quantity. There is nothing left to prove in the way of sexual attractiveness or prowess, but only a lifelong relationship to enjoy!

During 1990, women in this country endured 49,000 facelifts, 79,000 eyelifts, and 81,000 collagen injections! How sad that women in their forties and fifties are still trying to achieve the youthful appearance which appeals to the younger man, while misunderstanding completely the more complex picture of what sexually arouses the more mature man. Would you like to know what excites your man? Here's the secret, at no extra charge: confidence in your relationship, as expressed in the willingness to be sexually relaxed and innovative. Trust us, he's not interested in counting wrinkles. Your lifelong, unwavering commitment to him is a total and complete turn-on. Our concept of sexy beauty desperately needs to be redefined in terms of intelligence, warmth, commitment, character, and integrity.

I never have had a strong sex drive, and I have doubts that I'll become a sexual athlete at this point in my life. Is there something wrong with me?

Human sexuality is a unique experience; there is no minimum requirement for libido. A couple's level of sexual activity is a deeply personal matter, which will vary during the course of their marriage. It may need to adjust to all sorts of circumstances, and hopefully it will mature and improve with time. Ideally, sexual interests, likes and dislikes, and attitudes can be discussed between husband and wife—although there is, unfortunately, often great difficulty verbalizing these issues.

Problems can arise from a variety of areas, one of which may, indeed, be a discrepancy in levels of interest or desire. Most often (but not always) a husband desires sex more often than his wife. If you're wondering whether this will last forever, keep in mind that your husband may "mellow out" later in life, especially if his testosterone levels decline. And remember that 23 percent of menopausal women report an *increase* in libido; so if your sex drive hasn't exactly set records up until now, you might be pleasantly surprised. In fact, eventually you might reach the same place in desire for frequency.

But the emphasis was never meant to be on the frequency of sex. Sexual pleasure is the icing on the cake of a committed, loving relationship. Some couples are simply content to replace the sexual intensity of their earlier relationship with more satisfying nonsexual activities, and less frequent but satisfying sex. (It's called "companionship," folks.) In healthy relationships, the later years often focus on the sensate pleasures: holding hands, touching, hugging, and holding.

This vision of long-term sexual bliss sounds nice, but what if the sexual component of a marriage hasn't been good for years? How in the world could menopause and aging make things any better?

As we noted earlier, this very intimate aspect of a relationship often is the one a couple is least willing to discuss, let alone seek help for. But it's never too late to enter into counseling—hopefully together, but by yourself if necessary. If you need to discuss your own sexual issues, you can seek out a female Christian therapist who is comfortable with this area. (We would not recommend bringing this topic to your pastor, unless he and his wife together are co-counseling you and your husband. As wise as he may be, ventilating in private to a pastor about such a touchy subject is fraught with potential complications for both of you.) Very often a sexual disturbance in marriage is the symptom of other, more far-reaching issues which need to be explored in an appropriate setting.

During her years of counseling, Teri has come to realize that a majority of women—Christians in particular—are extremely guilt-ridden and confused about their own sexuality. For a society so focused on the free expression of libidinous urges, far too few people know the first thing about enjoying the full range of leisurely sexual intimacy.

One of the primary reasons for this deficiency—aside from unhealthy notions with which we were raised—is that too many Christian women have never developed a confident sense of their identity in Christ. When we fully grasp that we are God's beloved, that he created us with wisdom and love, and that he endowed us with incredible capacities, we cannot be defined by anyone's standards but God's. Sex and pleasure are not human inventions; both were designed by God as part of who we are. To deny our sexuality is to deny God's gift, to call "unholy" that which God has called "holy." The freedom that comes from this revelation spills over into all areas of our lives.

If this has not been your experience, a good counselor can take you through the difficult but very worthwhile process of dealing with guilt, so you can truly begin to live as the whole person you were intended to be. If you are unable to find or afford appropriate counseling resources, you can obtain a great deal of information and insight from reading. Unfortunately, much of the material you might find at the local bookstore assumes a worldview and moral standards (or lack thereof) that are hostile to biblical teaching and even common sense. We would highly recommend the writings of Cliff and Joyce Penner, especially *The Gift of Sex*, as resources which are not only thorough but also respectful of the ground rules given to us by the Creator of sexuality.

I'm already into the menopausal process, and I've never experienced more sexual desire in my life. It's embarrassing! What's going on?

Remember—in the Stanford Menopause Study, 23 percent of postmenopausal women reported an *increase* in their sexual desires. That's a sizable slice of the pie, especially since it flies in the face of societal expectations. But there are several plausible reasons for this change. First, some women experience a rise in androgen levels following menopause, although this cannot be universally correlated with sexual interest (see below). Second, the fear of pregnancy has disappeared, allowing woman to relax and enjoy sexual contact more fully. Also, there is more privacy in the house, no fear of the kids barging in. And, finally, many women are just simply less tired now that the years of childrearing are behind them. All things considered, there's no need to be embarrassed. Your husband might be pleasantly surprised by the change.

I read an article recently about testosterone replacement therapy to improve libido in menopausal women. What can you tell me about that?

Very little, as the research is relatively new and the jury is still out on this issue. Just as men have small amounts of estrogen on board their hormonal systems, women's ovaries produce small amounts of testosterone. Unfortunately, ovaries used to be routinely yanked out during a hysterectomy (the old "while we're in the neighborhood" procedure), but we now know that postmenopausal ovaries *continue* to produce androgens (an array of male hormones, including testosterone). There is much research in progress on testosterone supplementation, especially for women who have had their ovaries removed.

But this is also an issue on a broader scale, because some research also suggests that estrogen replacement therapy reduces our levels of testosterone by as much as 30 percent. This could raise a few sticky questions regarding HRT's interference with the sex drive. As we said, the research is too new to draw conclusions. One major problem is that the "ideal" level of testosterone for women has never been established, and too much of this hormone, as you might expect, leads to heavy facial hair and lowering of the voice—probably not an ideal scenario at this time of our lives.

I have been sexually abstinent since the death of my husband six years ago, but I am anticipating remarriage in the near future. Is there anything special I should do to prepare for sexual intercourse after such a long hiatus?

It would be a good idea to have an exam, including a check of the sexual equipment, to make sure you won't encounter any unsuspected discomforts. In particular, if it appears that you have developed atrophic changes, this would be a good time to consider some estrogen supplementation (either topical or body-wide), assuming you are postmenopausal and haven't done so already.

Another major annoyance to discuss with your doctor is the so-called "honeymoon cystitis," a bladder infection involving bacteria that the vaginal tract hasn't seen for a while. This is not just a problem for young brides. Anyone who begins having intercourse after a prolonged period of abstinence is at risk for cystitis, and the menopausal woman is especially susceptible. Most women have experienced the discomfort of cystitis at least once in their lifetime (the constant urge to urinate, then it hurts when you do!) and know that it responds quickly to medical treatment. Some doctors will prescribe a "preventive" dose of antibiotics for the honeymoon. Fortunately, cystitis usually will not recur if sexual activity remains somewhat consistent.

Do you have any last words of wisdom?

We're really glad you asked, because here's our parting shot: Perhaps you were raised by a mom who didn't know how to talk frankly about sex, because *her* mom came straight out of the Victorian era. In fact, when you consider that Grandma's attitude about sex was probably formed around the old adage, "Just lie there and think of England," it's pretty amazing that Mom was able to choke out anything at all! During a round table discussion of menopause, one woman in her mid-fifties quipped, "When I was first married, all my older friends told me sex was going to be horrible and I wasn't going to enjoy it. After I tried it I thought, 'What's wrong with me? I *like* it!'" In addition, many of us were raised in religious atmospheres which, unfortunately, instilled the message that sex was dirty rather than implanting the correct proposition that sex is created by God, beautiful, exciting, and meant to be reserved for marriage.

Sexual response is a learned behavior, and it's *never* too late to be a student. If you never received straightforward, factual information about sex when you were younger, it's not too late to start. At fifty, you are *not* over the hill—you're only beginning to reach the crest. Sex is *not* the random contact sport that the media so often presents. It can and should be an unhurried time of intimate communication between two people who have been longtime companions on the same road. After all these years, isn't it time you relaxed long enough to explore these pleasures—maybe for the first time in your life?

Chapter Nine

Is the Best Yet to Come?

What do you want to be when you grow up?

I thought I was asking the questions.

For this final chapter, you don't need to. This is a coda, a send-off, a pep talk before the big game. Sit back and relax for a few minutes, because after we're done you'll need to get to work.

If you're like most women who are approaching menopause, or already past it, you have probably buried that question for years. What do you want to be when you grow up? Did you think there would be no life after diapers and bottles and chauffeuring and scouts and piano lessons and parent-teacher conferences and graduations? Well, think again! Remember: women now live an average of thirty years after menopause. You have as many or more years after the kids are gone as you spent raising them. Did you think these years were destined for wearing out rocking chairs or (worse) remote controls?

What is your image of what an "older woman" should be? It is vitally important to review your role models for the middle years and beyond because you will unconsciously begin to imitate them. If your mother and grandmother, for example, endured menopause and beyond as though they were medieval martyrs, chances are that you may be expecting a similar fate. Decide now to change the mental video tape which equates menopause with dumpy bodies and frumpy dresses, because we have a way of making choices that match that internal image.

Menopausal women have traditionally served as the butt of many a comedian's monologue. They have been characterized as depressed, emotionally unstable, sexless, hysterical witches to whom everyone had better give wide berth. How did this stereotype develop? It is based on very limited experience, to be sure, because only the last couple of generations of women have lived long enough beyond menopause to create any kind of image at all!

If your mom was part of the post-war crowd of young wives and mothers, her emotional landscape was shaped by an era where everything was concentrated on rebuilding the nation and family. There wasn't much time for personal development or contemplation. When she hit the menopause years, her only model was her mother, who was probably ailing at sixty.

Whenever Teri looks at old pictures of her mom, she is always impressed by how much better her mom looks now, compared to thirty years ago! Teri's mom is a prime example of a woman who threw away the ridiculous stereotype of the postmenopausal woman and who took advantage of her new-found freedom to provide leadership to a women's ministry, accept speaking engagements, develop friendships, and pursue beauty.

While you're settling into your menopause orbit, you

might want to grab two or three good friends who are also starting this process and start your own informal "Menopause Survival Support Group." One woman we interviewed confessed, in amazement, that she and three close friends had silently dealt with menopausal symptoms for several months before one of them finally brought it up at lunch. From that time forward, they talked about it openly—commiserating, praying, and mostly laughing with each other. Until that time, each woman thought she was going crazy. "I'd go to the doctor with my long list of symptoms and sound like a hypochondriac!" Together they did their own research on menopause and educated themselves and their husbands. "The key is educating yourself about your hormonal life," one woman stressed. "There's such a variety of opinion in the medical community; we need to become experts regarding our own bodies and take some responsibility for the outcome." Amen!

If a mid-life emotional crisis takes place, it is likely to be a crisis of identity. "Now that the kids are gone, who am I? And do I want to find out?" The woman who has figured this out a little earlier in life will experience a much smoother emotional transition during the menopausal years. Unfortunately, the majority of women spend twenty to twenty-five years giving everything to their families, with little time spent figuring out what they want to accomplish after the job of childraising is over. This contributes to an unceremonious arrival at the forty-fifth or fiftieth birthday, feeling old, tired, used up, and lacking direction.

We spent a good deal of space in Chapters Four and Five discussing some emotional and spiritual aspects of the menopausal process, and we recommend you go back and re-read this material. In many ways, it contains the most important messages in this book. We believe it is impossible to sustain deep peace and contentment throughout the aging process without understanding who you are in relationship to the Creator. Just as a parent would gladly sacrifice any possession, donate an organ, or even give up life itself to save a dying child, so we have been redeemed from eternal death by a Creator who loves us more than any earthly parent could ever demonstrate. As our body continues on its inexorable path toward physical death, our worth can only be understood in terms of the parent-child relationship we have with God, and the wonderful promise that, because of Christ's work on the cross, we will eventually be wrapped with a new, ageless body.

We believe that a lot of mid-life emotional distress is derived not so much from physical changes as from a lack of preparation, stemming from denial. The beginning of mid-life wisdom is to acknowledge that our youthful period is over. It's time to strip down, turn on the bright lights, look into your mirror and say, out loud, "I earned every one of these lines, pounds, and stretch marks, and I'm proud of them!" Are you still secretly comparing yourself to the body of a twenty-five-year-old? Give it up! There is a beauty (and, yes, even sexual appeal) which emanates from the inner glow and self-confidence of an older woman who knows her worth.

While some may lament that youth is wasted on the young, the reality is that with the wisdom of many years comes the body of many years. Your goal is not to cling frantically to the ridiculous idea that you can retain youthful looks, but to revel in the fact that you have abandoned the absurd notion of worth based on appearance.

This may be particularly difficult for the woman who was derailed sexually during her younger years because of sexual abuse. The survivor of early molestation "learned" that her worth was inextricably wrapped up in her ability to provide sexual gratification. If this concept is not corrected at some point, the aging process will be especially difficult because her sense of value will disappear with her youthful looks. If you were a victim of sexual abuse and have never shared this secret or dealt with the shame and anger attached to it, this is the time to find a Christian counselor or mature friend, and then begin to understand the true basis of your worth.

The ability to create is a major part of what defines us as women. While fertility is the most obvious expression of that ability, our creativity continues long after the reproductive years have ended. We continue to create through those we now influence and guide: not only our own children and grandchildren but also other younger women in our sphere of influence. We also continue to create through our ministry and volunteer opportunities, through our hobbies, through an expanded or even first-time career, and in a thousand other ways which are now available because of the gift of time that has suddenly been given.

If you are near retirement from a job outside of the home, the coming years should be a time of new agendas, not terminal boredom. (This is sometimes more difficult for men, whose sense of worth is generally centered on their occupation.) Paul's mom, who worked from the time her children were in high school until her husband's retirement, is positively flowering in her seventies. (We have always envied her energy and wished we could borrow even half of her dynamism.) With the responsibilities of work and her own childrearing far behind, she has blessed us with years of loving "grandchild-care," countless wonderful meals, and attention to hundreds of little details which have beautifully facilitated a smoother family routine for us. Far from the stereotype of the interfering mother-in-law, Teri has found her to be an extraordinary role model for loving childrearing. In addition to the positive influence she has had on our family life, Paul's mom has also developed a new and very active role leading an auxiliary group which raises funds for a family camp ministry in Southern California.

It's never too early, or too late, to develop a vision. The

first part of your life is coming to a close—so how do you want to spend the second half? Start with taking stock of what you've accomplished so far. Some of you will be pleased with this review, while others may find it depressing. If you're discouraged, this is the time to meet with a counselor and seek to understand how you made your choices and how those choices (along with other events out of your control) may have derailed your vision of how your life would turn out. If seeing a counselor is impossible for whatever reason, grab a friend who is going through a similar review and work your way through a recovery workbook such as *When I Grow Up ...I Want To Be an Adult* by Ron Ross (Recovery Publications, San Diego, Calif.). If you've spent the past two or three decades tending to the family, you may not have the slightest idea how to begin developing a vision for yourself. What were your passions when you were a young adult? This is your chance to dust off those long-forgotten dreams and pick up where you left off before a pile of daily responsibilities crowded them out.

We already spent a good deal of time extolling the virtues of returning to school for the purpose of mental stimulation, so we won't harp on it now. But we do want to reemphasize that a first or a different career (one that you enjoy, this time!) can be started at this point in your life, if that is the direction you choose. If you're completely clueless as to what might interest you, ask a local high school or college career counseling office to administer a simple pencil-and-paper vocational test to help you pinpoint possible careers.

The last point we want to make in this closing chapter is that you can move into your final decades with the confidence that there is a place for the wisdom you have accumulated over the years spent on this earth. Paul, writing to Titus, said: "Teach the older women to be reverent in the way they live ...to teach what is good. Then they can train the younger women to love their husbands and children, to be self-controlled and pure..." (Titus 2:3-5). Too many young women are starting marriage and childbearing at a distance from their extended family. Without the benefit of older women guiding them past the hurdles of married life, career choices, and spiritual development, they are left stranded in the quagmire of moral anarchy which currently dominates our culture. Reach out to someone who is walking the road behind you.

Is the best yet to come? Absolutely. Menopause is not the end of your life. It marks the end of one era, but it can also signal the beginning of a personal renaissance. Such transitions always provide the opportunity for real growth and change. This is your turn in life, and if you're willing to do a little internal housekeeping, preparation, and self-education, the coming years truly will be the best of all.